I .... . UK

Charles Schoenfeld and
A Funny Thing Happened on My Way to the Dementia Ward
Memoir of a Male CNA

"In a humble, compassionate and humorous way, Charles Schoenfeld helps us understand that even when Alzheimer's steals every single memory, there still remains a person who is capable of being loved. "A Funny Thing Happened On My Way To The Dementia Ward" is required reading in the caregiving course we teach at Western Oregon University. Students appreciate learning how to connect with and care for people who are living in a reality that is very different from our own. Tender, poignant and laugh-out-loud funny, this book is a must read for families and professionals who are caring for individuals with Alzheimer's and other forms of dementia."

Elaine K Sanchez and Dr. Alex A Sanchez
Co-founders of <u>CaregiverHelp.com</u>
Salem, OR

"Reading a book that I know will end but don't want it to......Great book."

Pauline Baker
London, UK

"Best money I have spent on a book in years. I did not want this book to end."

Jen Wilson
Lake Ozark, MO

"...reading your book I went through just about every emotion. It is true and honest, real, informative, funny, sad, beautiful, all wrapped in one. Several years ago I ran the medical record department for a convalescent hospital, so I have been around plenty of people with dementia and Alzheimer's. When this terrible disease attacks a loved one, it is even more difficult.

Your book is exactly what I needed at this time. Thank you for your servant's heart and the reminder that no matter how awful this can be, there are still so many blessings. I cannot help but to wish you could take my dad hunting. At this time in his life—he would be in heaven!"

Shawn Brooks
Smyrna, TN

"I recently retired from working as an LPN in nursing homes for the last thirty years and have collected stories along the way with the intent of somehow letting people know of the life that goes on in those places, as opposed to the usual stories that get printed about them.

I believe CNAs are the most under-appreciated group of workers we have in our society. They work their butts off routinely doing jobs that would repulse, wear down or frighten their fellow citizens and as they do these jobs you can feel the love that flows from them to the persons they care for.

You did exactly as what is called for in seeing the residents as unique. Your remarkable creativity in divining what would be helpful to salve the souls of your residents needs to be recognized and put into action in homes nationwide. I am hoping to hear that someone in power reads your book and recommends you as a consultant to Wisconsin homes that show interest in putting their money where their mouths are. Once they see the results I believe the word will spread like wildfire."

Dorothy Tucker, LPN
Saint Paul, MN

"This has to be the most heartfelt book I've read concerning such an ugly disease. Charles writes with humor and love. I feel like I was there with him, getting to know his charges. I was moved to laughter, and to tears, as he told of his time as a caregiver. When/if I ever go down that path myself, I want a 'Charles' in my life. These people's lives were richly blessed by your presence, Charles."

Charlotte Bamsch
Georgetown, TX

those struggling through circumstances and makes them laugh along the way. That is why this book is a rare and wonderful gift to readers who have been waiting to hear from Charles Schoenfeld. He has written a real winner!"

Susan Engebrecht
Author/Columnist of articles for inspirational, literary and environmental magazines, including *Chicken Soup for the Soul* books
Wausau, WI

"I love Charles' book! The honesty of his stories make you laugh; the emotions of his stories make you cry. Literally, I was laughing one moment and then would have tears rolling down my face. My husband didn't know what to think! Charles was our Keynote Speaker at our 2013 Caregiver Conference in Fond du Lac. His true emotions came out while he enlightened us with his stories....he had us all hooked from the start. Many conference attendees listed him as the best part of the conference. He's changed many people's lives in the simplest way...by caring."

Michele Wix, CMA (AAMA)
President/Owner
Above and Beyond Care Solutions, LLC
Fond du Lac, WI

"Your book was in my mailbox today, I started to read it, I didn't want to put it down, but I had to finish some of my Christmas Eve duties. When I picked up for the 3rd time I couldn't put it down, When I was chuckling to myself (my family was looking at me weird) I was laughing with tears running down my face, I teared up, then I was crying with rivers running down!!! Thank you for reminding me why we do the things we do!!!"

Tara Nellessen CNA
Eland, WI

"I'm sure there are folks who wonder how you could find anything funny about dementia, but we who deal with it know that there are many times when without a sense of humor we'd all crack up! Charles is a very loving, compassionate man who writes of his patients with great respect and affection. I found the book valuable in that it just reminded me to appreciate the sweet things about my husband and to keep focusing on the positive. I loved what Charles said describing his job: "This job enlisted me in a war that promised no victory. The most I could hope for was to serve honorably until the end." That is my hope as well."

Karen Downing
Belpre, OH

A Funny Thing Happened on
My Way
to the
Dementia Ward

MEMOIR OF A MALE CNA

BY
CHARLES SCHOENFELD

Charles Schoenfeld

Acknowledgements

The events in this book are real. With the exception of my family and co-workers, names have been changed to protect individual privacy.

For the past six-plus years I worked on a nursing home dementia unit. This book is dedicated to the individuals with Alzheimer's I helped care for, and to all who suffer dementia.

Thanks to Lori Koeppel, Janice Baron, Kristin Woller, and the lady from the State of Wisconsin who granted me a Nursing Assistant license. All had faith my good would outweigh my bad. Thank you Cagney Martin, a giver in a world filled with takers. Thanks as well to Merry Wimmer for her diligent research while dealing with my incompetence. My gratitude to Ann Brooks for her friendship and insights, to Sue Engebrecht, for her mentoring and encouragement, and to Chari Fish for her skillful editing efforts. My deep appreciation to those who allowed photos to be included in this work. Finally, to my wife, Maggie, who put the pen in my hand and insisted.

Author's Note

There are bridges to cross in every life. Most of us proceed with caution, concerned about the waters below. We've heard stories of those who fell and vanished, never to be seen or heard from again. On occasion though, someone once thought lost is discovered on higher ground, cleansed and renewed.

Many of us reach a time when we grow tired of tiptoeing or trudging along, fearing any slip or unforeseen gust of wind. At that point, there is only one option left – a leap of faith. This book is about caring for those living with Alzheimer's, though I'm not someone with diplomas on my wall. Nor am I a tormented son lamenting a loved one's fate. I'm a man who was doing just fine, though growing tired of a life spent marching by in locked obedience and harmless obscurity, as so many of us do, when suddenly I found myself standing at cliff's edge. Since that day I've learned the true rewards of life are waiting for anyone willing to seek them. I didn't know it at the time, but this book was born the day I decided to jump.

I haven't produced an epic, I know, but it's what I had in me. When you're someone not really educated, not really a writer, you end up with something long on effort, short on volume, and an author questioning his own sanity. This writing is not a research project or a classroom attempt to assist someone looking for answers. It's what I experienced, and how I felt and dealt with those experiences. Others working beside me may have seen things in an entirely different light.

Introduction

Nursing home care in America has a dubious history. In the early 1900s, with no Federal assistance available, most elderly and disabled people were sent to poor farms, or "almshouses." These facilities were dilapidated; the care was poor and inconsistent. When the Social Security Act was signed into law in1935, it provided grants to each state through the Old Age Assistance Program. People living in almshouses however, were not eligible.

This opened the door to the concept of private, old-age homes, allowing elderly citizens to live where they could receive care, while also collecting assistance payments. It wasn't until the 1950s that amendments to the Social Security Act required nursing homes to be licensed. Money was made available for the construction of new homes, modeled after hospitals. Instead of being part of the welfare system, homes were now in the health care system. For years following, nursing home scandals were uncovered, revealing financial mishandlings, along with non-compliance of code and staff requirements. Federal programs came and went. In 1987, the Omnibus Reconciliation Act, "OBRA," directed the largest-ever overhaul of nursing home regulations.

Today, teams of State and Federal regulators arrive unannounced to conduct nursing home inspections. The inspections last several days, and include all aspects of nursing home functions, from diet and personal care to record keeping.

During one such inspection in April of 2009, North Central Health Care, Wausau Wisconsin, was found to be one hundred percent in compliance, an extraordinary accomplishment. Recently, NCHC achieved a Five-Star rating, ranking it in the top ten percent of nursing homes in the United States.

*"A man's real possession is his memory.
In nothing else is he rich, in nothing else is he poor."*

Alexander Smith

The Asylum

I was walking outside with a resident at 2:00 p.m. on a mid-July day when a hospice nurse approached me with the news.

"Charles, I'm so sorry. Your mother has just passed away."

I'd gone to see Mother a couple of hours earlier. A hospice employee was giving her a sponge bath, so I didn't enter the room. I heard her groan softly, not realizing it would be the last time I would ever hear my mother's voice.

I hurried to her, reciting every prayer and last good-bye that came to me, as if promptness might still allow me to reach her.

You might think such a moment would cement itself into your memory forever. For me, it has become a blurred recollection that carries a certain amount of guilt. I should have slowed down. When something needs to be done,

I tend to rush and lose all attention to detail. It's a trait I got from my mother.

Around our house, my wife, Maggie, handles everything. Her role in our relationship has always been that of the pod and mine, the humble, needy pea. I've got all I can do to water the lawn and answer the door. Now, however, Mother's services and estate were my responsibility. Even though I knew this was coming and had planned for it, I was still caught off guard. Everyone forfeits a life. The big question, when is payment due? It would have been much more convenient had this happened in one of those far-off tomorrows.

I drove to the funeral home to make arrangements, then headed back home, my mind busy with phone calls to be made and documents to be located. Two blocks from our house, I noticed nursing home employees peering behind bushes and searching through the wooded area down towards the lake. I realized instantly that someone had wandered away from the facility. Right then, though, I really didn't need the distraction; my plate was already full. Nevertheless, I found myself joining in the search.

It took perhaps ten minutes to find who we were looking for. A gentleman in a motorized wheelchair, a past stroke victim, had simply decided to go for a drive. When I found him, one side of the machine's wheels had left the sidewalk and gotten stuck in a stretch of mud. He was still seated, unable to extricate himself, the chair tilted at a dangerous angle. I got to him and kept him safe until help arrived.

It wouldn't have been a big deal on an ordinary day, but I was in an emotional state of mind, melodrama pumping through my veins. Was what just took place a circumstance choreographed by my mother to demonstrate there was still a need? Mother's situation had led me to the nursing home in the first place. Once her time there ended, I had assumed mine would be ending as well. This turn of events changed things. If there was any possibility Mother was sending a message, it was something I couldn't ignore. I stayed on at the nursing home.

Standing on the sidewalk in front of my house and looking to the west, I can see North Central Health Care. That nursing home was the last place I saw my Aunt Alice.

Shortly after getting out of the military, I drove Uncle Ron there to visit her once a week. Despite living in the same town, I was never close to my aunt and uncle, probably because they never had children. Aunt Alice was a tiny thing who loved her martinis. At family gatherings she always had one in her hand, although that one drink lasted her all night. She'd peck at it like a bird, barely wetting her lips.

I had been away in the Air Force for four years and didn't know how long she had been at the home. She was no longer able to talk. Instead, she mumbled rapidly and I couldn't make heads or tails of what she was saying. My uncle sat with her while I hung in the background, not knowing how to act.

She wasn't walking anymore and the home had fastened a board to her wheelchair, which acted as a table. She shuffled a deck of cards over and over, never playing any games. Walking towards the exit after our visit, we'd turn for a final look. Aunt Alice would still be shuffling those cards. It strikes me, now, how alone my uncle must have felt. A helpless wife, no children, and no longer driving on his own had changed his world.

During colonial times people who suffered from mental illness were thought to be possessed by the devil. They were dealt with accordingly. Treatments included "ice baths," rendered until the patient lost consciousness, and "blood letting," the removal of "bad" blood. Many died. By the early 1800s English asylums used a rotating device in which the patient was whirled around at a high rate of speed. Mental health care's darkest hour in America may have arrived in the 1930s when Dr. Walter J. Freeman introduced the trans-orbital lobotomy. This procedure was an actual "separating" of the brain. Two quick shocks to the head provided sedation. At that point, an upper eyelid was lifted and a shaft inserted. The shaft was tapped with a hammer until the desired depth had been reached, then wiggled back and forth. This part of the procedure was the "separation" process.

I had little knowledge of the facility where Aunt Alice stayed. When I was a kid, the place was referred to as The Wausau Insane Asylum. The name itself made me want to keep my distance. Built in 1893, the official name was Asylum for the Chronic Insane, and the total annual cost for housing a resident was approximately one hundred dollars. Today that amount probably wouldn't see a resident through breakfast. It's possible if you close your eyes and whisper, "Asylum for the Chronic Insane" you'll be visited by a vision of Alfred Hitchcock.

The original facility housed upwards of three hundred people. About the same number reside in the nursing home today, although the current facility is much larger. The original home was considered a model for its time, but must have been considerably overcrowded. In 1893 no one wanted to know what was going on behind those locked doors. Even now, over a century later, most of us prefer to look the other way when it comes to facilities devoted to diseases of the mind. This book is my attempt to shine a light into that darkness and give you a peek inside.

When I first entered the dementia and Alzheimer's unit, I carried the same unwarranted fears, stigmas, and personal misconceptions that many others harbor. They were tucked in my pocket for safe keeping, ever available to remind me this was something I didn't have to do. I wouldn't be blamed if good intentions crashed head-on into reality. I learned things had changed since the days of Dr. Freeman. What I discovered waiting for me there, instead, was a lesson in humanity.

Someone in the United States develops Alzheimer's every sixty-nine seconds.

CHAPTER 2

Mother

Family legend has it my great grandmother was kidnapped by Indians, never to be seen or heard from again. It was an event that prompted my grandfather to load his wagon and leave the small village of Petit-Rocher, (Little River), New Brunswick Canada, and head south. He ended up settling in Tomahawk, Wisconsin, forty miles north of Wausau, where he eventually found work with the Post Office. One hundred years ago the mail arrived daily by train. Grandpa would start his day at the depot, unloading, sorting, and eventually distributing mail to the carriers. With an average of eight bags of mail arriving each day, he used a push cart to accomplish his work.

As the town and volume of mail grew, a horse and wagon were needed. Grandpa not only built the wagon, he owned the horse, Rosie. The mare resided in his back yard. Whether it was a job he loved, or simply endured, is hard to say. Grandpa wasn't prone to sharing his feelings.

My memories of Grandpa are mostly of a large man sitting on his front porch, comfortable in a wooden rocking chair, smoking a pipe. Retiring in 1953 at the tender age of eighty-five, he lived to be ninety-four, and passed that longevity gene on to many of his nine children, including my mother, Florence.

Mother was a real estate agent who spent most of her time selling houses to herself. We never moved up, just over. By the time I was eighteen we had moved a dozen times. Dad's patience with her seemed limitless. She promised each move would be our last. Then, just as we were putting away the final few boxes, Mother would burst in and proclaim she had finally found the perfect place.

When Dad died, Mother remained a widow for the rest of her life, a time span of twenty-seven years. She spent most of that time moving and eventually found her way to a retirement mobile home park in northern Wisconsin. During the next six or seven years, I moved her into four different mobile homes within that same park.

We finally coaxed Mother into renting an apartment in Wausau near Maggie and me the year she turned ninety-four. Her stay at that apartment lasted about a year, and it was tough duty. I checked on her every morning before work, and Maggie stopped by in the evening. It became increasingly apparent that Mother could not live on her own. There was no specific, glaring problem that needed to be addressed, but her ability to care for herself was diminishing.

After a good deal of coaxing she agreed to come to live with us. When I stepped into her apartment for a final check of the place, I immediately fell flat on my face. She had washed the kitchen floor with Crisco oil. She had that floor so clean you could cook off of it, and that's how things were beginning to go with her. She knew she wanted to leave her place clean but was a little off-center as to how to go about it.

Mother spent three half-days each week at an adult day care program at the nursing home. The rest of the time she was home alone while Maggie and I worked. I came home one evening to find her sitting in her chair, her face and blouse covered in blood. How I got through that moment without a heart attack remains a mystery. She looked dazed but explained that she had tripped and fallen while taking a walk and "the lady" brought her home. The blood was from a nose bleed, but we never learned who the lady was.

More than a year later, I discovered that the woman who would one day be my boss at the nursing home had also been the Good Samaritan on Mother's behalf. Mother had walked to the K-Mart store about a mile from our house. She was returning home toting a couple of shopping bags when a drenching downpour began. My future boss was driving by when she noticed an elderly woman standing on a corner, forlorn and soaking wet.

The only thing she recalls Mother saying to her was, "Please don't tell my son."

Maggie and I were sitting with Mom one evening, voicing our concerns about her well-being during those times when she was home alone. Mother reassured us she was capable.

"Don't worry about me. If anything happens, I'll just call 91."

After nearly a year with us, we put Mother on a plane to Texas, where she would spend the winter months with my sister, Jean. While she was enjoying the southern warmth, Wisconsin was going through an old-fashioned winter. Mother became concerned about the strain deep snow would cause to the roof of her home and dialed the park manager. She asked if it would be possible to have the snow removed. He assured her the matter would be taken care of and the cost wouldn't exceed seventy-five dollars. Mother didn't hear well on the phone but believing the job was within her budget she immediately sent payment; a dollar bill and a note, "Keep the change."

While in Texas, she fell more than once. When she returned in the spring, she was in a wheelchair. One of her falls had broken a hip. She was ninety-seven and had reached the point where we could no longer provide the care she needed.

For most people a nursing home is a last resort; a place to remain as safe as you can, and as comfortable as you can, for as long as you can. No matter how justified a person might feel in placing a loved one in a nursing home, there is a burden of guilt that doctors, nurses, social workers and clergy cannot ease. My brother and sister both live far away. The task I had always dreaded but knew would someday rest with me, had arrived. On May 3, 2003, we moved Mother into North Central Health Care, the nursing home down the block.

Alzheimer's and dementia caregivers had $7.9 billion in additional health care costs in 2010.

CHAPTER 3

Leap of Faith

Many of today's nursing homes make an effort to create a home-like environment, focusing on each person's individual needs and background. North Central Health Care is a large facility catering to a wide variety of needs. The nursing home is referred to as Mount View. The name alludes to the sight one is treated to at the rear of the building. It sits on a high bank overlooking Lake Wausau. Beyond the lake to the west rests Rib Mountain. The Rib is no Mount Everest, but it is the highest skiable mountain in the state and has bragging rights as the second highest vertical drop in the Midwest. Lake Wausau is a bit less than two thousand acres in size, an offshoot of the Wisconsin River. The river provides the city with a kayak course that hosts racing competitors from all over the globe.

Mount View Nursing Home sits on a parcel of land that I'd guess is close to sixty acres. The grounds are tree-lined and groomed. A paved walkway circles the entire perimeter and has strategically placed benches. Though the Home is located at the edge of a residential neighborhood, it's not at all intrusive. People walk and jog around the building's walkway. Children's soccer matches take place on the expansive front lawn.

We've always liked it here. The first home Maggie and I bought was in this same neighborhood, five or six blocks from where we live now. A retired couple in their sixties lived behind us. One night a ruckus outside awoke me and when I went to investigate, I found my neighbor in his underwear, climbing on my woodpile. Days later, Maggie rescued him from the K-Mart store where he was wandering around, gathering items in his arms. He'd left his car running in front of the store entrance. One of the store managers followed him around, not quite sure what to do. Luckily, Maggie happened in and volunteered to help. She drove Bill home. His wife had called the police after realizing her husband was not in the house. She tearfully confessed that there had been problems for quite some time. She'd been taking care of him by herself, trying to keep their circumstances secret.

Other than Aunt Alice, my neighbor was the first person I'd ever dealt with who suffered from Alzheimer's disease. There was no way for me to know I would deal with hundreds more.

Mother settled in at the nursing home as well as we could have hoped. Most of the people living on her end of the building were elderly and in situations similar to hers.

Occupational, Physical and Speech Therapy are also housed there. A long passage called the link hallway connects the nursing home to the Behavioral area of the building, where Dementia Units C and E are located. Upper D Unit is home to a wide variety of people, some who may have dementia; most with psychological problems that severely limit their ability to function in the community. Lower D is a short-term acute psychiatric unit. These residents may have been brought here because they threatened to harm themselves or others, or because of the ramifications of drug and alcohol abuse. Many arrive by squad car.

There is also a staff break room, a kitchen and cafeteria, a beauty shop, a dentist office, and a lab for blood work in this area.

Patients with developmental disabilities have an area of their own. Some are dropped off each day by loved ones; others are escorted by group home workers or arrive by bus. They spend the day here "working." Around mid-afternoon they are picked up and returned home. Adult day care where we used to take Mother is here as are two gymnasiums and a swimming pool. Sprinkled in and around are a multitude of offices and other programs that serve the community.

I stopped to see Mother every morning before heading to work and visited again in the evening. She was on a lot more medication due, in part, to her hip injury. In my judgment, it contributed to her diminished reasoning. She liked to invite people in to "see her place." "Her place" was one room which she shared with another lady. She had a single bed, a chair from home, a television, and some family pictures. In retrospect her frame of mind was probably a good thing, but it did little to ease the guilt I felt for having brought her here.

In late July, Mother contracted a severe urinary tract infection. It was devastating. Her entire system began to shut down, and she was no longer eating. Soon she was hospitalized, and the staff did their best just to get ice chips in her. Mother was still lucid and able to talk, even chipper

at times. She seemed unaware she was in a battle for her
life.

Knowing our mother couldn't go on like this forever,
my sister, Jean, flew in from Texas. In my opinion, her
arrival saved Mother's life. Jean was the favorite and seeing
her only daughter gave Mother an immediate boost. Jean
is a great cook and began making homemade soups, just
broths at first. It began with a sip or two, then a couple of
spoonfuls. After that, it was game on and pass the chicken.

The nursing home staff was more than a little surprised
to see Florence come back. When she left for the hospital
things had been looking pretty dire. But the trauma of the
past few weeks had taken a toll. Her aging mind and body
had burned up a lot of resources. She began to wander
off the Unit, forcing staff to search for her. There was real
concern that she would one day find her way outside. Then
what? C unit serves people with Alzheimer's; there are more
eyes to watch over things. Doors have alarms that alert staff
whenever someone is leaving. As her things were being
carted down the hall, I knew my mother was moving for the
last time. It was a move that would change both of our lives.

Mother was not perfect, which explains why she didn't
raise a perfect son, but I do know any virtues I carry with me
were learned in the home she provided.

I continued to visit daily, a task made easy by the facilities
close proximity to my own home. I admit to being a little
intimidated my first couple of visits. A dementia ward is a
place the average person would need a little time getting
used to. Whenever possible I tried to arrive at meal time,
bringing a favorite snack for Mother and visiting while
she ate. During meals she was always seated at a table with
three other residents. At first I tried to ignore them but
soon learned that was not possible. How do you ignore

someone using the wrong end of a spoon? To my surprise, I found myself enjoying everyone's company! Here was a place where nobody put on airs, worried about saying the right things, or gave a crap about how your kid was doing in school. In short, I'd found somewhere I fit in.

Two people at the table were no longer capable of feeding themselves, so a Certified Nursing Assistant or CNA, was always there to help. On one occasion when the CNA was called away for a minute, I took over where she had left off. After all, I'd seen it done dozens of times. When she returned, she informed me politely that what I was doing was against regulations. I was a bit miffed but beyond that, rather pleased at the good feeling that came over me for having performed this small task, even if only for a minute. I have a nature that some might describe as a bit unusual, and I wouldn't argue that. But in this environment, it seemed to suit me well. The residents at the table clearly began to like me. If one was having a bad day, I did my best to comfort, but most of the time we laughed. Laughter is the best medicine.

I retired from my driving job with United Parcel Service on October 3, 2003, the day before my fifty-sixth birthday, with twenty-seven years to my credit. Now I have a readily available answer when I hear the phrase, "What can Brown do for you?"

I drove directly to North Central Health Care. The next CNA class was due to start November 19. I realized that trying to go from truck driver to Alzheimer's aid would be making quite a leap but I had a gut feeling. So I jumped.

Fifteen million caregivers provide seventeen billion hours of annual unpaid care valued at $202 billion.

CHAPTER 4

Class

In general, I've always found learning a difficult proposition. When I was young, I didn't understand old people. Now I'm older, and I can't fathom young people. For thirty-five years of my life I've been married to two different women. Not at the same time, that would be crazy. I've raised a son and three daughters. Yet I still haven't figured out the women. I know its imperative I be a good listener. They like stuff that's soft, and eat a lot of lettuce. After that, things get murky. Not that marriage is bad for a man. In fact, I've reached the conclusion it's a good thing. It teaches virtues a single guy would lack; things like patience and obedience and how to be content when suddenly doing without. Did I mention being a good listener?

Years ago I may have been a wise guy, but now I just say, "Heck yeah! Try on as many as you like!" "Yes dear." "No dear." "Maybe tomorrow night" and, "Could you repeat that? I had the game on too loud."

I've never been much of a student either. That blame lies squarely with my parents. Mother's first husband was killed in a car-train collision. By the time she met my dad and remarried, they were both well into their forties when I came along. With time an enemy they did their best to hurry things up. I was the youngest in my grade school class and in my high school class as well. Do you know what it's like to feel rushed? To not quite measure up to your peers?

While classmates were starting to grow beards, I was waiting for baby teeth to fall out. When those same guys were picking up girlfriends in their fathers' cars, I was still contemplating the willing consumption of my first vegetable. It was a horrific situation to be in. While in high school the legal drinking age in Wisconsin was eighteen. Not for hard liquor, but there were "beer bars." Our state's leaders decided the hard stuff was off limits but saw nothing wrong with young people gagging on a barrel of suds. While my classmates were out at these establishments making fools of themselves and throwing up in back seats, I was at home on the couch eating popcorn and trying to keep my eyes open until the ten o'clock news. Now I'd gone from that scenario to this; from the youngest to by far the oldest.

There were nine of us in the CNA class, eight cheerleaders and me. I thought if I failed this class they might hire me as a chaperone, or possibly to lecture on the importance of birth control. I'd just put my fifty-sixth birthday behind me, so I wasn't hard to pick out. I was the old one, the bald one, the one without a hickey on my neck. The term feeling out of place doesn't begin to describe me.

Our instructor, a female nurse who would later quit to pursue a promising career in Amway sales, thought it would be a good idea if we all got to know each other better. To that end, we each took a turn at the front of the room and talked about ourselves. I wanted this to work, but killing myself now seemed a viable alternative. I listened to stories of love, love lost, of boyfriends, fiancés, furry pets of every description, and the numerous times something happened that was really, really funny. After awhile my mind drifted off to a place that begged the question, *what in the hell am I doing here?* However, the girl sitting directly in front of me, who could have made millions doing acne commercials, told us about her two thousand dollar coon dog that had been attacked and killed by wolves. She even had pictures! *Her* I listened to! I'm much more comfortable with the outdoor theme.

When it was my turn to speak, I stood mortified in front of the class. I didn't have a clue about how to begin, when a girl raised her hand with a question.

"Are you a psychiatrist?" Obviously it hadn't occurred to her I might be a classmate.

"No, I'm a retired truck driver." I went on to explain that "retire" is something you do after you have worked somewhere for a very long time.

At break time, everyone had a diet Mountain Dew in one hand and a cell phone in the other. As if on cue, everyone dialed, or punched in, or whatever it is you do with cell phones to get them activated. I won't drink pop unless it's mixed with something that burns my throat, and I don't own a cell phone. Who would I call? Maggie?

"Hi Sweetie, just wanted to hear your voice."

She'd think the cheese finally slid off my cracker. Besides, not having one helps cut down on my listening time.

I stood there, hands in my pockets, jiggling change and considered the possibility of clipping my garage door opener to my belt, just to fit in. I didn't really want to call anyone. I just wanted to give the impression I could if I wanted to. These phones must come with a set of instructions that direct the owner to start every conversation by asking, "Whatya' doin'?" This appeared to be the common thread anyway.

The phrase "and I'm like" was used constantly. "He said he's breaking up with me and I'm like," or, "So now everyone leaves and I'm like…" Where was I when that started? There is a lot of meaningless babble until finally a "love you too" brings an end to each conversation. With three breaks a day and thirty days of classes, I witnessed this entire process ninety times.

Once the calls had been completed, my classmates interacted, but I wouldn't describe the subject matter as intellectual. Most of it ran along the lines of why Madison's sister called her a slut, favorite pizza toppings, and who got the drunkest last Friday night. They did make short mention of skin cream products and movies I knew I never wanted to see. It's as though I'd somehow been beamed into an episode of *Grey's Anatomy, The Early Years*. The saying goes, "If you want to get nowhere, just follow the crowd." From that first morning forward, the search was on for empty hallways.

From time to time, we left the classroom for various destinations throughout the building. It usually had to do with a particular piece of equipment we needed to become familiar with, or to witness a demonstration of something we'd need to be able to do ourselves one day. Our instructor led us down the hallways, where I knew we stuck out like sore thumbs. Everyone we passed recognized us as the new kids on the block. I straggled as far behind the group as possible, convinced anyone casting even the slightest glance in my direction said to herself, "Look at that old bald guy, the one without a hickey."

There was some structure to the lessons we learned but overall, our instructor ran a fairly loose ship. She liked to encourage discussion, and opinions bantered about included topics that ranged from abortion to reincarnation. One large girl near the front was a legend in her own mind. She sported a rose tattoo on each ankle, the flowers far beyond actual size. I assumed they were scaled to the girth the artist was dealing with. Were those thorns sticking out, or leg hairs? It's apparent early on that she was the alpha female and someone worth avoiding. I found myself at odds with everything she had to say. Even her breathing started to bother me. I would dearly have loved to form a rebuttal and bring some reality to her gibberish, but why muddy the waters? I was too intimidated anyway.

In the end my classmates agreed unanimously that they are against abortion. I heard a lot of "my body is a temple" sentiments. Regarding the alpha female, I couldn't quite make that connection, but I was in agreement with views expressed. I didn't believe in reincarnation, but then I didn't believe in it during my last life either. I've surmised our instructor pursued this format with the hope that a certain amount of bonding would result. At break time I bolted for the door and searched for places to be alone, glancing over my shoulder to make sure I wasn't being followed.

I'd been in classes for barely a week and was still trying to settle in when the facility hosted a party for nursing home residents and their families. Maggie, my two youngest daughters and I were excited to bring Mother. The event was held on the beautiful patio area behind the building where everyone could take in the view while enjoying free food and music. We were seated at a table with a man in a wheelchair who was struggling to feed himself. Outgoing and pleasant, he told us he was a farmer and a life-long bachelor. A stroke had landed him in the wheelchair and brought him to the nursing home. Throughout the meal he was talkative and friendly, even sharing a joke or two. Though he would have had every right, he never demonstrated any bitterness regarding his circumstances. Once he'd finished his meal his face was streaked with mustard and ketchup along with a dollop or two of baked beans. Though my CNA classes had just gotten started I'd come to realize there would be much more to my job than simply sitting and clowning around with the residents. This poor man's face needed cleaning and I was seated nearest him. I heard my voice say, "Let me help you." I felt like I had ten thumbs as I wiped away each stain. Through the thin napkin I could feel the sharp bristle of another man's whiskers. No doubt most people would have done what I did and regarded it as a matter of little consequence. But to me, with my family there, it was a "Look what Dad can do" moment. He smiled and thanked me and I sighed with relief. In that instant the truck driver in me vanished. Suddenly I was one hundred percent certain; I wanted to be a caregiver. In the years that followed I helped care for hundreds of dementia patients and confronted the myriad of challenges they presented. When it was all over and I was ready to retire for good I'd learned one rock-hard truth. The greatest obstacles I ever had to overcome had been my own insecurities.

∽ ∾

As my classes continued some of the skills we learned included how to reposition someone who is bedridden, correct ways to assist with feeding, and how to use a hoist for lifting someone who is immobile. We measured a person's liquid intake and output and learned how to record that information. We were taught the correct way to take a person's pulse and practiced this new-found skill on each other. I was teamed with a skinny nineteen-year-old who took my pulse first.

"Sixty."

Then I took hers.

"One hundred twenty-two."

I wanted what she was smokin'. I assumed they'd teach us CPR, but we never got into it. I supposed practicing chest compressions at "Camp Cleavage" could be problematic. I was older but not dead! We learned a myriad of basic do's and don'ts when dealing with dementia. Do validate what they are saying. Do use a sense of humor. Do praise and encourage. Always approach from the front. Don't argue. Don't try to reason. Don't give orders. I learned dementia is not a disease in itself, but a symptom. Sort of like someone who sneezes may be coming down with a cold, dementia suggests abnormal thinking. There are over one hundred causes of dementia, with Alzheimer's suspected in sixty to eighty percent of cases. Then we got down to the nitty-gritty and the point where my confidence started heading south: bathing and toileting. These two tasks, especially toileting, take up the greatest part of a CNA's workday. Suddenly, bailing out was an option worth consideration. During those visits with Mother around the dining table, talking and joking with the residents, was what I had enjoyed. For those residents whose dementia was beyond that type of interaction, I felt empathy and a desire to comfort. Wipe their butts? Not so much.

There was a dummy we practiced on. I don't mean a dull-witted person, I mean a kind of manikin. It pulled double duty. One minute it was a male, then tugged hard in the right place (this part always gave me the shivers) it was good-bye Wally, and hello, Sally. Even at this I was a nervous wreck. It didn't help that my classmates giggled in the background. Every time I stepped up to that damned dummy, I felt my face flush. My breathing would be labored, and my mind would go blank. At the first opportunity, I took my instructor aside and confessed that I really wanted to work here, but I simply could not stomach the personal care stuff.

At that point, we had one girl who simply quit. I gave her credit. We were paid $8.00 an hour to take this class. She could have milked it, hung in there until the classes were finished, and then walked out. My instructor told me not to be concerned, that it's a big place, they'd find a spot for me somewhere.

However, she added, "You'll still need a CNA license, and you'll still need to finish the classes." Feeling somewhat reassured, I stayed the course. Various assignments and written tests were not the problem; it was just that damn dummy! The fourth or fifth week in, a day I had been dreading arrived. We left the classroom and the dummy behind, and headed for the front line – bath day. Each of us would be given the opportunity to demonstrate the skills we had learned on a real, live, breathing, in-need-of-a-bath person.

Walking down the hallway, my classmates laughed and talked, as if on their way to pizza and a movie. Meanwhile, I struggled through a personal nightmare that grew worse with each step. The only thing my seizing brain was able to pass along to the rest of me was, *OH GOD, OH GOD,*

OH GOD! It turned out not to be a bath, but a shower. To me, that was about the difference between a firing squad and a beheading. Each of us had our own resident and our instructor there to help us along. That reassurance brought not one ounce of comfort. An elderly woman was brought in wrapped in a blanket. About this time I started feeling faint. I watched in amazement as one of my classmates actually volunteered to go first. I wanted to go last. Maybe I would get lucky and the world would end before they could get to me.

Suddenly, the nurse turned to me and asked, "Chuck, are you ready to jump in?"

I wanted to tell her I'd prefer to have my fingernails pulled off with pliers, de-vein a boat load of shrimp, root for the Vikings. You can throw in ant problems.

Do it for me, and I'll give you my house! OH GOD, OH GOD, OH GOD. Trembling with fear I heard my own voice betray me.

"Well, of course I'm ready."

My resident was a male. I couldn't make up my mind if that was a good thing or a bad thing. I took a deep breath and held it, closed my eyes and stepped in. Before I knew it, I was on my hands and knees, searching for those hard to reach spots. *What did I just touch? OH GOD. OH GOD. OH GOD!* Water pouring over me helped to distract my panic stricken brain. Time stood still while I gasped for air and scrubbed ever so gently. In self-defense my mind had wandered off to a place far, far away when mercy finally arrived. A tap of a hand on my shoulder, and it was over; I'd done it!

At the end of our six weeks, we needed to pass the Clinicals test in order to receive our CNA license. A former nurse, now working for the State, was brought in to conduct this procedure. Each of us would randomly select a piece of paper from a bowl. Each piece of paper had three tasks we needed to perform correctly. Eight of us were tested, with each test lasting about fifteen minutes. We waited in the hall, and one by one we were called in for our exam. When finished, we were advised to return to the hallway and wait. Our instructor of the past six weeks would bring us our results.

The nervousness I felt waiting in the hall paled in comparison to entering the test room and spying that damned dummy. I got my set of instructions from the bowl. The first was range of motion exercises. No problem. Second, assist with feeding. *This is so easy!* And third, a bedridden female resident (that damned dummy) has had a bowel movement. Assist with personal care. I felt my face flush, my mind went blank. I labored to breathe.

Minutes, or was it hours later, I found myself back in the hallway. I hadn't a clue what had just transpired. Not long after the last student had been tested, our instructor showed up with the results. She was smiling; everyone had passed.

Well, not quite everyone. The State lady wanted to talk to me. My heart sank, and I'm sure the disappointment showed on my face. She made no comment about my performance, but had one question.

"Why do you want to be a CNA?"

I wasn't kidding now and hoped she could appreciate the sincerity in my voice. I told her about Mother, my frequent visits, and the residents I had met, that I knew I couldn't do personal cares, but surely there must be something......
I just wanted to help. She thanked me, and I was excused from the room. Back in the hallway, the waiting was agony.

What will I do if this falls through? What will I tell Maggie?

I'm not sure how much time passed before the nurse found me. She gave me a hug.

"Congratulations, you passed."

The next day I was informed that I had been assigned to E Unit with the job title DTA, Dining and Transport Assistant. My hope of being a caregiver was about to become reality and I could not have been happier. Starting pay was $7.88 an hour, a twelve cent an hour cut from what I'd been paid to attend school. *What the hell's up with that?*

According to the Alzheimer's Association, 26.6 million people worldwide suffer from the disease. In the U.S., 5.3 million. Unless a cure is found, by the year 2050, these numbers are expected to quadruple.

CHAPTER 5

E Unit

Twenty-six people lived there. Considerable effort is put into making E Unit as homelike as possible. It's basically one big room. The dining area is equipped with tables and chairs to accommodate everyone at meal time. There are tablecloths and centerpieces. The remainder of the room is carpeted, furnished with couches, recliners, and a large round table for socializing. There is an oversized television, a piano, and at the far end of the room, floor to ceiling windows offer a view to the outside. The bedrooms are around the circumference of the room, the majority with two beds per room. A small staff bathroom is tucked away in a corner. There is a tub room where residents are bathed and a quiet room with sensory items for calming.

On the wall a large message board proclaims: THE MONTH IS DECEMBER-THE WEATHER IS COLD-THE NEXT HOLIDAY IS CHRISTMAS. E Unit also has its own kitchen equipped with a stove, refrigerator and microwave.

Finally, there is the nurse's station. The walls are made of glass, allowing anyone working inside the ability to keep an eye on things.

No one, including my boss, knew exactly what a DTA was supposed to do all day. They'd never heard of the position, much less had one assigned. The focus of my duties was to assist at meal times and to accompany residents when they left the campus for things like doctor appointments.

After a brief tour and a few introductions, I was left wondering what to do. The CNAs were going about their business, while the office staff was busy getting ready for the arrival of a new resident.

New residents "are like a box of chocolates, you never know what you're going to get," to borrow a quote from Forrest Gump. Some come in like a lamb. That day, we could hear the roars approaching down the hall as dozens of anxious eyes focused on the doorway. I'd envisioned this day being informative, but somewhat laid back. A little time to get my feet wet.

The wide-eyed charge nurse needed one second to issue me my first set of instructions. "You watch her!"

The rest of my day was a collage of *One Flew over the Cuckoo's Nest, Mission Impossible,* and *Rocky.* My patient's name was Mabel. She made her way around with the aid of a walker, which doubled as a weapon. Her repeated requests for the intervention of law enforcement officials to rescue her could only be described as ear-piercing. I tried, without success, to get her seated without breaking some "thou shall not restrain" rule. It wasn't long before *I* was the one hoping the police would show up. I obviously would need more time to master "redirecting," a key element taught in class when faced with unwanted behaviors.

"Tell me about your family Mabel. Ouch!"

"Look at the squirrel! Ouch!"

"Please, don't undo those buttons. Ouch!"

"Okay, but you're gonna catch cold! Ouch!"

"Mabel please, it's my first day! Ouch!"

I'd hoped to learn a lot that first day, but went home confident of only two things:

Mabel was not wearing a bra, though in my opinion a bra would have been beneficial. I really mean that. And she had a sneaky left jab.

The charge nurse had doubts that I would last on her unit and didn't try to hide her skepticism. With a confident smirk she suggested that if the people living here didn't get to me, the people working here probably would. Not so much the CNAs, who were grateful for any help they could get, but the office staff was another matter. The place had its cliques.

Being the only male, it wasn't long before the arrows started flying. By that time in my life I was pretty well insulated from the baldie remarks, but when they turned their attention to my age, the arrows stuck a bit deeper.

"We'd like to take you shopping, so we can get the senior citizen discount," was a frequent remark.

They were only having fun but it was a new arena for me, and I didn't handle it very well. I was a veteran. I'd been the Union Steward at UPS, raised a family. I felt disrespected. Maggie told me to ignore it. I tend to over think sometimes, but half of me believed that my boss's prediction might turn out to be correct. Meanwhile, my other half was discovering the residents. They opened my heart and jumped in. I quickly realized there was no way I would leave this place anytime soon.

There is something unsettling about being uncomfortable around your peers but perfectly at ease with people who aren't sure what planet they are on. On my days off I found myself back at the nursing home, clowning around with my new friends. They were children masquerading as senior citizens. Alzheimer's had thrown their lives into reverse, systematically robbing them of a lifetime of memories and lessons learned.

In class we had studied different parts of the brain and the purpose for each. The hippocampus is important to memory and learning. It's the first part of the brain to be affected by Alzheimer's. The temporal lobe controls thinking. The frontal lobe determines personality, mood, and behaviors. The occipital lobe, vision, and the cerebellum controls coordination. Nine major parts in all.

That's all nice to know but if I was to help, I had to stop trying to make sense of everything, be myself, and go with the flow. Knowledge is a good thing, but of little use when someone is pouring their milk on the floor. It became my experience, the proper solution in a situation like that is to quack like a duck. I settled in, and somewhere along the way the teasing from my co-workers stopped. Quack!

We were taught you can't bring a person with dementia into your world. You have to go inside theirs. It's 6:25 a.m. and a female resident named Bonnie is coming towards me as I arrive for work. I don't recall ever seeing her up this early, and have never seen her in her nightgown before.

Obviously upset, she yells to me, "Let the damn dog in!"

I turn around and whistle, then call "Here boy. Come on. Good dog!" Satisfied, she turns around and goes back to bed. I'm thinking this isn't rocket science.

Though I had found acceptance, I didn't do a lot of socializing. My social skills have never been honed, destined forever it seems, to a dull blade. I ate my noon meals in the cafeteria, usually alone. The food wasn't gourmet, but after thirty-three years toting a lunch box, it was a small luxury, and the food wasn't bad if you were really, really, hungry.

There were always announcements in the break room about upcoming parties. Avon, Amway, Tupperware, knick-knack-patty-whack parties. This was a world I never knew existed and I steered clear. When it came to my feminine side, I had to draw the line somewhere. Not wanting to seem totally standoffish I made an effort to form a mud-wrestling club, but the concept never gained a foothold.

Mabel's stay with us lasted about five years. Hers was an agonizing battle. Dementia, mini-strokes, infections. Finally, her body had just had enough. It would not be truthful to say we had a lot of fun together. Dementia or not, personalities vary. Some folks I could do all kinds of silly stuff with and we had a great time; others I could not. Mabel was someone I just wanted to keep calm. If I accomplished that, she enjoyed a good day. The nursing home found medications that helped, but even then she could be difficult. Still, we had a lot of conversations and I took her on many walks.

There were two occasions with Mabel that are most memorable. The first was a beautiful summer day and my day off. By then Mabel was in a wheelchair. I went over to the nursing home and brought her over to my house, wheeling her onto my deck in back. I had prepared a lunch I knew she would like. The grass was green, the flowers blooming. I turned on the sprinkler, and soon robins were hopping around looking for their next meal. It was quiet. The beauty of simplicity so often overlooked by a world in too much of a hurry. Mabel's speech was limited by then, but she managed to say the only thing I needed to hear.

"It's so beautiful."

For a couple of hours, a troubled mind found peace. It was one of those times after which you crawl into bed at night thinking it had been a good day. And you sleep well.

The second occasion wasn't so much about Mabel, but the fact that she was with me at the time. It was 7:00 p.m. on a Friday evening. I'd be off work in another hour. Bedtime approached for many residents, so we tried to set the mood. Radio and television volumes were turned down, lights dimmed. I might have been passing out a snack, or giving someone a back rub, but normal activities were done for the day.

Mabel began yelling. She had it in her head that her sister was supposed to pick her up. They were going shopping, her sister hadn't shown up, and—

"Where the hell's my sister?!"

One loud person can stir a chain reaction, so I took Mabel for a walk off the unit. All the offices were closed, the halls empty. She was still hollering for her sister when we rounded a corner and saw a man in a wheelchair headed our way. I recognized Billy, who lived on Upper D, a unit with some stunningly interesting people.

Billy has been on Upper D a long time, and was granted a certain amount of freedom. I never knew when I might see him cruising around in his wheelchair. He's in his fifties, although he looks to be younger. The shape of his body always reminded me of an egg, in a Humpty Dumpty sort of way. He seldom used his hands to wheel himself along, preferring to stretch his feet out in a walking motion.

Over the years Billy collected an amazing assortment of fireman hats, police hats, FBI badges, and military insignia. A lot of his stuff looked real. How he accumulated everything was a mystery. In his mind he had served his country in every branch of the Armed Forces. When he

informed me one day that he was an Army General, I asked
how many men were under his command.

"Fifty," was his reply.

I surmised that recruitment must be on a down turn.

Here's the thing you gotta know about Billy. When he's
wearing a fireman's hat, he *is* a fireman. Everyone in the
building knows Billy. For the most part they played along
with his scenarios, but they could sometimes cause problems.
Once upon a time Billy landed himself a pair of genuine
handcuffs. He locked himself to a handrail, not realizing
he'd lost the key. It costs money to call in the experts.

When he wore a policeman's hat he cupped his hands
and spoke into them. He was now in contact with police
headquarters.

"Yeah, this is Billy. "Keek keeek" (he mimics static). "I'm
in the link hallway. Can you give me a description? Over.
Keeek."

Meanwhile, Mabel's lamenting had in no way diminished,
and sensing trouble, Billy inquired what the problem might
be. Mabel, relieved that someone was finally paying attention
to her predicament, tearfully belted out that her sister, who
was supposed to pick her up, had not arrived. Billy's hand
darted for his shirt pocket, where he retrieved a pen and
notepad. His now firm voice took command of the situation.

"I'm Billy with Building Security. How long has your
sister been missing?"

I rolled my eyes and shook my head, but Mabel was so
stunned she finally stopped yelling.

In addition to the hero thing he had going, Billy also
fancied himself a lady's man. It mattered little that the
object of his affection may be married with six kids. If the
lady was on his turf, she was fair game. His leanings in this
regard were not the least bit raunchy.

He wrote poems, for instance. If he met you in a hallway, he'd ask if you would be so kind as to deliver his "Roses are Red" message to the nurse, CNA, or secretary who had caught his attention that day. If not a poem, perhaps he'd request delivery of a trinket won at bingo. These were tasks I performed for him many times. Eventually a memo directed that we were not to encourage or enable Billy in any way with this sort of thing. An order is an order, but that's not to say I was in agreement. Billy enjoyed fantasizing about the female staff. *Didn't everybody? Were we the only two?* I've yet to meet the man whose moral compass arrives with a guarantee. Hell, mine's all over the place!

At bingo one day, another resident reached over and took a swig out of Billy's can of pop. Furious, Billy stuck his hands out like a grand master.

"I know karate," he warned. "I'll use it if I have to."

Billy eventually moved to a group home. One of the other male residents of Upper D grew tired of his bravado and punched his lights out. The karate apparently didn't hold up.

Whenever I think of Billy, I'm reminded of a line from Michael Perry's *Population 485*.

"Until courage meets consequence there are no heroes."

If it were that easy Billy, we'd all be doing it.

∽ ⌒∽

Being new to E Unit and to the job, I had a lot to learn and a lot of people to get to know. There was Jim, the hard-working little farmer, tough as a three dollar steak. Jim hadn't stopped working just because he lived on the Unit now. With a flip of his wrist he had a table turned over. On hands and knees, he changed oil and adjusted gears. There was never a shortage of work on a farm. To get him upright I'd plead, "Jim, its lunch time." or "Jim, you've got a phone call." I was wasting my time. There was work to be done and Jim was burning daylight.

He'd decide when it was break time and then recite the rosary.

"Holy Mary, Mother of God, Holy Mary, Mother of God."

There was Little Lila, with her perfectly round face and Coke bottle glasses. Add to that huge blinking eyes and a toothless smile. Remember the movie character E.T.? Stick some thick glasses on him and you had Lila. I used to ask if she was still in contact with the Mother ship. In order for her to hear me I'd have to shout everything into her left ear, repeatedly. A nursing home resident here since her sixty's, she was approaching one hundred years old. No one visited her and she hadn't walked in so long that her ankles withered to a circumference hardly bigger than my thumb. Yet she was lovingly feisty. Clamping her lips down on her gum line, she'd squeeze my finger and threaten, "I'll kill ya," then go back to chomping on the pureed sandwich I'd just given her.

And Emma, so devout. Her sister was a nun. To get her to eat I would summon my deepest voice.

"This is God speaking, Emma. Open your mouth."

Then there was pretty little Nellie, just a wisp of a thing. Every day she told me about her son. How proud she was.

"He's a helicopter pilot, flying secret missions for the government." She couldn't tell me much about it, it was all very hush-hush.

Nellie loved snacking on chocolate chips, the kind you put in cookies. The family brought them in by the ton. We served them to her in small Styrofoam cups. Late afternoons were hard; something would come over her. She would start to shake in her recliner, almost as if the chair were vibrating.

"Help me-Help me-Help me," she'd chatter, machine gun-style, sliding out of her chair. All the while it would rain chocolate chips.

I was so gullible back then. Desperate to get to know and help each resident, I'd hang on every word.

Maria had suffered a stroke and could no longer walk. When she tearfully confided to me she knew she could walk if only the facility would provide her with some therapy, I ran to the nurse with my discovery. I was feeling rather self-righteous. *For God's sake, the least we can do is give this poor woman an opportunity.* I was informed that Maria had been here for years and during that time had received therapy scores of times.

Roberta was another lady who tweaked my sympathetic tendencies. She was always claiming something of hers had been stolen. The list of missing items was interesting. A chicken, a pig, her fur coat, but in most cases, money. The amount never varied, it was always six thousand dollars. She suffered shortness of breath, managing only a few words at a time. Each burst of words would be louder than the last. A sentence that started out in a normal tone would be a scream by the end.

"I can't...believe...someone stole...my six thousand...dollars!!"

I spent a lot of time trying to console her and brighten her day in any way I could. Again one afternoon she was missing six thousand dollars and knew exactly who the thief was. Me! I was crushed.

"You can't be serious. Me?!"

Alzheimer's transforms the strong to the weak. By all accounts, Big Bill was well known and respected in his farming community. His adoring family is testament to the person he'd been, and the kind of life he'd led. They brought in a picture of Big Bill, circa World War II. He was a young Marine at the time with wavy brown hair and a chiseled chin, an image perfect for a Marine recruiting poster. In the picture he's laying in a hospital bed. Wounded but smiling, he's shaking hands with Eleanor Roosevelt. Another picture, taken years later, hung on the wall in his room. It showed Bill walking across a field on his farm land, hand in hand with a tiny grandson. Cupped in his opposite hand, with no more apparent effort than one might apply to hold a golf club, Bill toted a tree trunk. A gentle giant, tireless provider, with an indomitable spirit, now laid helpless by an enemy that doesn't care. For Bill's loved ones, his condition was a torment that would not sleep.

So yes, I met a lot of people, and became increasingly aware of the suffering endured by others.

When I was a young man my perception regarding anyone with dementia or a brain injury was quite different.

I heard about Junior, a guy who went to a different high school, and had a rough and tumble reputation. News traveled fast in the circles I was entrenched in at that time in my life.

"Did ya hear about Junior?"

"Yeah, crashed his bike huh?"

"Yeah. Guess he's a vegetable."

"Yeah. Wananother beer?"

At the time of that conversation, I was probably in my late teens. Starting work on E Unit nearly forty years later, I learned that a long-time resident had recently passed away.

At one time in his life he had enjoyed riding motorcycles. His name was Junior.

I've learned to recognize my blessings.

The risk for developing memory problems that may signal early Alzheimer's seems to escalate after age fifty. Nearly eleven thousand baby-boomers are now turning fifty each day.

CHAPTER 6

That Time of Day

Agitation. Catastrophic "exaggerated" reactions. Wandering. Sundown Syndrome. Rummaging and hoarding. Repetition. Inappropriate sexual behavior. A list of only a few of the symptomatic behaviors that I became familiar with.

Inappropriate sexual behavior is something I'd seen little of. Perhaps because of the disparity in our male to female population – six men to twenty women. Whatever the reason, I remained eternally grateful.

Of all the disturbing behaviors, Sundown Syndrome was especially interesting. It's a phenomenon that occurs in mid- to- late afternoon, affecting some residents more than others. For those who are affected, the change in mood and personality can be dramatic.

Bonnie was someone I mentioned earlier, the lady who demanded I let the dog in. Bonnie was agreeable and pleasant, but at exactly 4:00 p.m., a transformation took place. Suddenly angry and distrustful, she hurled accusations and struck out at the staff. She might list any number of atrocities that had been forced upon her. No amount of apologizing or attempts to appease her did any good. We kept play money in the nurses' station for Bonnie, as we were often accused of robbery.

Maria was another example of Sundown Syndrome. Usually quiet and satisfied early in the day, by late afternoon she began complaining.

"I want to go home now."

As afternoon turned to evening, she became louder and more persistent.

"The bus dropped me off this morning. When the hell is it picking me up? I came with a group of ladies, now I can't find them! How long does this party last? I WANT TO GO HOME!"

She demanded we get her daughter on the phone. This scenario took place every afternoon, without fail. Maria had lived at the nursing home for eight years, and long ago her daughter asked that we no longer allow Mom to keep calling.

Showing Maria her room, her name above the door, the family pictures, her clothing in the closet and dresser did no good. It was all some kind of trick we were playing, and Maria knew better. She was someone whose speech was not affected by her disease. A stranger talking with her might spend a fair amount of time before realizing that something was not right. I was chatting with her one day when she unexpectedly asked if I had enjoyed my Christmas holiday. It was August at the time, so I needed a minute to think back.

While I knew exactly what to expect from some, with others it was always a surprise. Upon receiving a bag of popcorn one evening, a resident promptly went around the Unit tossing it all on the floor…feeding the chickens.

Tom was extremely unsteady on his feet but was always trying to walk on his own. I'd just reached him after seeing him get up when, grinning all the way, he stiffened his legs and began throwing his feet high in the air, marching around like an inebriated version of Hitler's finest.

∽ ∾

Something I'd noticed about the nursing staff was how unflappable they could be, especially when things were topsy-turvy. The longer I was there, the more I tried to follow the example they set. Getting Alzheimer's patients to take their medications, often several times a day, was no easy task. Just getting someone to open his or her mouth took skill and knowledge of the person you were working with. Once that was accomplished the pill, or pills, still had to be swallowed, and kept down, something that seldom happened. Some residents refused their medications altogether, requiring the nurse to make repeated attempts. These nurses always hung in there with a can-do attitude, never appearing as frustrated as I knew I would be.

There is a mandate that I believe comes from the State, requiring that a person's medications be temporarily reduced from time to time. I assume it's an attempt to see if medications prescribed in the past may no longer be needed. Getting people off of unneeded drugs is a good thing, but the results of those efforts were usually immediate and dramatic. I shiver to think what it must have been like when the medications we now have were not available.

I had Dementia Specialist Training, classes given by the Alzheimer's Association. Along with the training was a lot of reading material, most of which I've kept. Today, research is making strides against Alzheimer's disease. One of the papers helped demonstrate that just one hundred years ago, efforts were in their infancy. The paper was titled, "The Perplexed Woman." The grammar was peculiar, but it is copied here exactly as it was written.

A fifty-one year old woman showed jealousy toward her husband as the first notable sign of the disease. Soon her family noticed a rapidly increasing loss of memory. She could not find her way around her own apartment. She carried objects back and forth and hid them. At times she would think that someone wanted to kill her and would begin shrieking loudly.

In the institution, her entire behavior bore the stamp of utter perplexity. She was totally disoriented as to time and place. Occasionally, she stated that she could not understand, and did not know her way around. At times she greeted the doctor like a visitor, and excused herself for not having finished her work; at times she shrieked loudly that he wanted to cut her, or she repulsed him with indignation, saying that she feared from him something against her chastity. Periodically she was totally delirious, dragging her bedding around, calling her husband and her daughter, and seeming to have auditory hallucinations. Frequently, she shrieked with a dreadful voice for many hours.

Because of her inability to comprehend the situation, she always cried out loudly as soon as someone tried to examine her. Only through repeated attempts was it possible finally to ascertain anything. Her ability to remember was severely disturbed. If one pointed to objects, she named most of them correctly, but immediately afterwards she would forget everything.

When reading, she went from one line into another, reading the letters or reading with a senseless emphasis. When writing, she repeated individual syllables several times, left out others, and quickly became stranded. When talking, she frequently used perplexing phrases and some periphrastic expressions (milk/pourer instead of cup). Some questions she obviously did not comprehend. She seemed no longer to understand the use of some objects.

Her gait was not impaired. She could use both hands equally well. Her patellar reflexes were present. Her pupils reacted. Somewhat rigid radial arteries, no enlargement of cardiac dullness, no albumin. During her subsequent course, the phenomena that were interpreted as focal symptoms were at times more noticeable and at times less noticeable. But always they were only slight.

The generalized dementia progressed however. Four-and-a-half years after the disease was first noticed, death occurred. At the end, the patient was completely stuporous, she lay in her bed with her legs drawn up under her, and in spite of all precautions, she acquired decubitus ulcers.

The paper's author was Dr. Alois Alzheimer, writing the birth of Alzheimer's research. While today's medications can aid in fending off unwanted behaviors, the eventual outcome remains unchanged.

Of the ten leading illnesses causing death in the United States, Alzheimer's is the only one that cannot be prevented, cured, or even slowed.

CHAPTER 7

The Fair and Farewell

Back on E Unit, I was getting better acquainted with the neighborhood and its inhabitants.

As nicely as I can put it, Eileen was no trip to Hollywood. A few inches taller and she'd have been the Packers' starting left tackle. Eileen was not aggressive; she just didn't know her own strength. For whatever reason she was not a big fan of moving. I'm not talking about Houston to Dallas. I'm talking about from this chair to that one over there. If left alone, there was no doubt she would hunker down in a recliner and remain there for all eternity. If your sport was lifting bolted-down fire hydrants, you'd love Eileen; but pull all you want, she wasn't going to budge. Trust me.

Her vocabulary consisted of one word, "chocolate," followed by a smirky giggle. It's what she said to me once she realized I was too tired to pull anymore. Like most women, she knew how to get what she wanted. We had a truck load of candy in the kitchen with Eileen's name on it.

One of the few times she moved on her own was when she decided she'd like to take a bath. It wouldn't matter that she'd had a bath an hour ago, or that the tub room was currently occupied. Giggling all the way, she'd pull staff members behind her like tin cans behind a wedding car.

Eileen didn't get many visitors but didn't seem to care. Who needed visitors when you owned the joint? Her reality was that I needed to give her chocolate. My reality was if I didn't hand over the chocolate, we had an overweight mummy in the green recliner.

She desperately needed exercise, but it was a Catch-22 situation. Before she'd agree to go for a walk with me, I had to hand her the standard bribe. I was hesitant to take her outside because she had health issues, and stamina was a concern. I also worried that if she took a notion, we might very well end up in Ontario.

Remaining inside, strolling hand in hand down the hallways, we were in a social setting that caused problems. Without warning, she would deliver a burp that was off the Richter scale, followed by her trademark giggle. I am absolutely convinced she did this out of a perverse need to see me humiliated, but that's not the worst of it. Some of the things I learned on this job I wish I hadn't. Women fart! Who knew? I'm not talking your garden variety oopsies. I'm talking about an every man for himself it's been good to know ya HELL'S TRUMPET!

Every head turned and despite being brought up a gentleman I wanted to shout, "IT WAS HER! WOMEN FART! THEY DO!"

I was left wondering if I'd stumbled on a category the Guinness people hadn't considered, as this had to be some kind of record. If I could bottle this stuff, I'd call N.A.S.A.

Eileen was among a group of residents we took to the County Fair, an outing we took every summer. I wasn't too concerned about her hallway antics surfacing. At a fair in Wisconsin she'll fit right in. Keep in mind that this is a State where, driving down the road, sooner or later you'd encounter a pickup truck with the moniker, "Gut Pile Lyle" emblazoned across the bug shield.

With all the residents in wheelchairs, we pushed our way past the rides, through the animal barns and into the bathrooms, where we spent the majority of our time. The real highlight of the day was treating everyone to some Fair food. Burgers with fried onions, corn dogs, fries, cheese curds and elephant ears. For dessert we had homemade pie. In Wisconsin we love our fests. October Fest, Brat Fest, I Remember Your Mother from High School Fest.

Eileen's a Wisconsin girl, so it came as no surprise, when someone handed her a can of non-alcoholic beer that she raised it to her lips and kept it there until the last drop trickled out. If you're of the notion this is something no woman is capable of, you've never been to Wisconsin. I get the impression that given the opportunity, she could keep this up all day. Just set a case in front of her – and step back non-believers.

We all backed up. She's gonna burp.

Our ventures to the fairgrounds provided many fond memories. Helping a person with dementia enjoy an ice cream cone in the hot summer sun provides enough material for another book.

On one Fair trip, we had an unusually high number of residents along - the result of several Units deciding to go on the same day. Someone was apparently operating under the assumption that I knew what I was doing and assigned me latrine duty. I was stationed outside the fairground bathroom to help any male residents that might need assistance. A female co-worker sat beside me to help the ladies.

As I sat upon that park bench under a warm summer sun, a gentle breeze caressing my face, I couldn't help but think there are so many ways this could go bad. In the three or four hours we were assigned, I may have had to assist one gentleman. Meanwhile, my poor partner barely had the chance to sit down. The line of women in need was never-ending. I was feeling relieved (Pun. I couldn't help myself) that I wasn't called upon more often.

My little security shell suddenly broke open when my partner came scrambling out of the lady's room insisting, "I need your help!"

Apparently, the wheelchair-bound woman she was trying to assist was not only a tad overweight, but lacked any leg strength whatsoever. It was going to require two people to get her out of the wheelchair and onto the pot. A sign taped to the back of the woman's wheelchair read, "United We Sit." An image I didn't care to contemplate. Still, I figured if I could grab an arm, lift, stare at the ceiling, hold my breath and pray, I could get through it.

There have been times in my life when I have felt out of place. This situation topped the list. I was in the women's bathroom at the County Fair! Granted, I'd probably been here before, but never when I was *sober*!

Surrounded by wide-eyed, gasping women cradling their daughters and reaching for their cell phones, I said the only thing I could.

"Trust me. I'm a Certified Nursing Assistant."

ᗦᎻᏂ ᏂᎻᗦ

Agnes was a cute hoarder. When getting her ready for bed at night, a table setting for four might fall out of her bra. If, from behind her bedroom door I heard a staff member yell, "Hey, I found my watch," I knew what had just happened. Hoarding is a common behavior for those with Alzheimer's. Maybe it's a person's response to a world they know is slipping away.

One of the first things we were taught is to never argue with a dementia patient. It's upsetting to that person, and there's no way to win. That being said, it could be tough. A co-worker told me about the day Agnes insisted the blouse the worker was wearing belonged to her. After an entire day of, "Give me back my shirt," the employee could take it no more.

"This is *my* shirt Agnes. I bought it at *Webco* for $12.99. I've got the receipt!"

Agnes was my best washcloth folder. We'd go through hundreds, maybe thousands of washcloths every day. Clean, rolled up washcloths were supplied to us in plastic bags. In order to get them distributed to residents' rooms, they needed to be straightened out and folded. Enter Agnes. Not everyone was capable of performing this task. For those who were, it not only provided something to do, but helped promote a feeling of self-worth. I'd break out the bags in mid-afternoon, a time when unwanted behaviors started kicking in. Keeping people busy was a way to offset those behaviors. Agnes was always front and center, and in no time would have a table full of stacked, neatly folded washcloths.

My problem now was getting them back. She'd lay claim to anything within reach, be it a washcloth or her neighbor's teeth. The fact that I was the source from which the washcloths first arrived was irrelevant. I'd try to act nonchalant approaching her.

"Hello there, Agnes."

I was just passing by, but she had an uncanny way of sensing what I was up to. The second my hand touched a washcloth, she'd latch on with the quickness of a cat, and the tug of war began.

"Give me them, they're mine."

"Thank you for folding these for me, Agnes."

"I want them!" She pulled harder now.

"For God's sake Agnes. I'm not after your virginity!"

At some point exhaustion forced me to quit and change tactics. Plans were put in place to create a diversion. When she was distracted, I swooped in and grabbed as many washcloths as possible before being detected.

Agnes had a way of talking where only her lips moved, all other facial muscles remained dormant. She was from Michigan's Upper Peninsula, so maybe the lip thing was something that evolved over time, her body's way of conserving energy when the weather turned brutal. There's a family picture album in her room that I've looked at many times. In the winter scenes, the snow is banked around her house as high as the roof line. When I approached her, I'd always get the same greeting.

"Cold, eh."

Its half question and half statement, and a phrase which most certainly originated during a northern Michigan winter.

Agnes had been a nurse, and the Peninsula's original First Responder. Both her daughter and her granddaughter became nurses. The latter works on this unit. As a First Responder, I can picture Agnes plowing her way through the mother of all blizzards on some U.P. back road, on her way to a farm where a boy's tongue is frozen to a manure spreader.

I see her then, bounding through the drifts, across the barnyard and up to the poor kid. When she kneels down, the first thing out of her mouth is, "Cold, eh."

When I arrived at work one day, I was informed Agnes had fallen and broken her hip. It marked the beginning of a downward spiral. Folding washcloths, her favorite pastime, ended. No longer accepting food, we relied on vitamin drinks, but they can only take you so far.

Her family had kept a chalkboard on the wall above her bed in an effort to keep her close. On it they listed names of family members, wrote down certain dates of significance, and special personal messages. Often when she was lying down I'd sit by her, reciting the messages and reading the names. Eventually they held no meaning for Agnes yet they continued to be written-and I continued to read them. It was one of many examples of how becoming a professional caregiver would weave me into the inner-fabric of other people's lives. A simple sign-off and signature on a card; "I love you Mom, your daughter Kate" takes on a whole new meaning when it's sent to a mother with Alzheimer's. This job enlisted me in a war that offered no promise of victory. The most I could hope for was to serve honorably until the end.

⁓ ⁓

I accompanied Kurt to the Eye Clinic downtown for his appointment. Although I informed the receptionist that Kurt was on medication and our window of opportunity was limited, the wait seemed to take forever. Once inside the exam room, things were still moving slowly when Kurt, silent until now, announced that he had seen people with their heads cut off. With that, the doctor suddenly located second gear. There was a point in time, early in his stay with us, when Kurt made remarks like that.

Nearly all of our residents were incontinent, including Kurt, but assistance with this chore was something he resisted. With his considerable size and frightening comments the female staff struggled with the process of getting him toileted and changed. At times he would not cooperate at all. Everyone knew how squeamish I was when it came to personal cares, but reasoning Kurt might be more comfortable with a male assisting him I was eventually asked to help out. Most often I'd hold Kurt's hands and do my best to make conversation while the girls went about cleaning him up. The sights, sounds, and smells during those occasions put my head to spinning. I tried my hardest to appear confident and professional as I drifted through a personal Twilight Zone. During my years at the nursing home I was asked countless times with numerous individuals to lend a hand with personal cares for a wide variety of reasons. As time passed Kurt's off-hand comments went away and his resistance to personal cares diminished. I, on the other hand, would never be able to overcome my painful, awkward ineptness.

Kurt had been a Surveyor and owned his own company. I learned he'd created Wisconsin's first statewide snowmobile trail map and once attended a snowmobile manufacturer's convention in Canada, making the round trip by snowmobile.

The family brought in pens, rulers, graph paper, all familiar items that Kurt could sit and busy himself with for hours. The work he produced was impeccable. Footages were noted, curb sites positioned, high water marks recorded. His penmanship was extraordinary. For a period of time he was back in the workplace, his confidence and self-worth restored. Eventually these skills would be lost, but for awhile they were a godsend.

He wandered into the kitchen one day where I found him tearing open tea bags and systematically dumping the contents onto the counter. I stated the obvious.

"Kurt, you're wasting all that tea!"

He let out a deep breath to demonstrate his exasperation, and replied, "Well I know that!"

Despite his considerable size, Kurt managed to sneak into the kitchen and climb out a window. It was the dead of winter with freezing temperatures, so he immediately climbed back in. Locks were then installed on all kitchen doors.

Kurt's wife has health problems of her own, and her mother has recently been admitted to Mount View Nursing Home. Yet she visits her husband regularly and never arrives without a smile for Kurt and the staff. I saw Kurt and his wife recently at the annual Valentine's Day breakfast. I sat with them awhile, not sure how many more opportunities I'd have to see the two of them together. He wore a brand new shirt his wife brought for him.

"Isn't he handsome," she beamed?

Kurt is no longer able to feed himself, walk or talk. Someone unfamiliar would have observed a smiling lady and a man with a blank stare at her side. How fortunate for me to know these people personally. It's a rare thing these days to witness true grit, and a promise kept.

෧෨ ෭෬

We had just gotten everyone seated and the breakfast trays passed out one morning, when someone behind me yelled out Eileen's name. Turning to look, I saw her face-down in her food, already turning blue. Gone.

We left her in her chair and carried her into her bedroom. From there, we lifted her onto her bed. After double-checking all vital signs, the nurse hurried off to make the necessary phone calls, leaving the rest of us in shock. I sent up a quick prayer. Outside the bedroom door, food was getting cold, the oblivious residents still waiting to be fed.

A minute later I was spooning pureed eggs into someone's mouth. Thirty feet away behind that bedroom door, a person I enjoyed and cared for lay dead. I wondered why the possibility of an event like this had never occurred to me. It wasn't mentioned in my CNA classes. I concluded that certain lessons can't be taught. They can only be learned on the job. We find ourselves laughing together one minute, crying together the next, none of us realizing how much someone means to us until we've lost them.

This is hospice moved up a notch. The ultimate win will one day be the discovery of a cure for Alzheimer's. Until then, taking a step, accepting a bite of food, or smiling in recognition, has to suffice. Pleasure danced with pain there all the time. I learned to appreciate the victories whenever and wherever I could.

∞ ∽

When a new resident arrived, we realized the person was functioning at the highest level we'd witness from them. There are medications that may help in some ways, but the wheels have already been set in motion. Things are slipping away. For example, when staff got someone up for the day, they'd offer the resident a choice of clothing.

"Would you prefer the blue pants, or the gray?"

A simple gesture helped provide dignity and an opportunity to let someone know that he still had some control over his life. At some point, though the staff might still offer a choice, it really wouldn't matter. The question had become difficult; too much had been lost. We noticed this in all areas of daily living, from diet and exercise to group participation. Alzheimer's can be like the proverbial snowball rolling downhill, forever gaining speed and dimension. While that may be the general rule, with some patients the disease progresses at a slower rate. Regardless of the pace, for anyone afflicted, their fate has been sealed, the only question being, "How long will this go on." I've always had a hard time fathoming the amount of destruction this disease inflicts on the human brain.

After a round of golf, I was sitting at the bar with John, a man I had just met. He asked what kind of work I did.

After I'd given my answer to him, he said, "Alzheimer's? That's when people forget stuff, right?"

It's hard to believe there are still people around with such a simplistic concept of Alzheimer's. What starts out as mild impairment will, over time, "unplug" the brain's ability to function. Legs and arms will no longer work. Reasoning will be gone. Eventually, the lack of nutrition will affect the brain's capacity to instruct the victim how to swallow.

I remember one example where Alzheimer's sucked every last drop from its victim, a woman who passed away soon after I started working at the Nursing Home. Her mouth had been open wide, while her body had curled into a tiny ball, as if in the womb. Her entire circumference

would have fit on a bedroom pillow. I don't remember her
making any sounds. If there were to be goodbyes to loved
ones, they needed to have been said years before.

---

*For someone with Alzheimer's, if no other serious illness
intervenes, lack of brain function will eventually cause
death.*

CHAPTER 8

Sally

The Alpha and the Omega. The beginning and the end.
The problem is ill fate often claims ownership to the
middle. I've watched as residents lay motionless in bed,
or lean backwards in a chair staring towards heaven as if in
a trance. Lila did that. Linda too. I'd like to believe they are
taking in the Wonder, but they seem bewildered. Had the
inequities they'd suffered left them questioning the purpose
of these lives we live. What were the tears and the hardships
of this earth all about? I didn't know what to tell them.

The resident with whom I developed the closest
relationship is the one who is the most difficult to describe.
It's finding words that are worthy of such a special lady. It
was an honor to have known her, and an absolute glory to
have been of help.

There had been a car accident and her husband did not
survive. Sally's many injuries were horrific. She could only
move her head and left hand and spent her waking hours
in a body-length wheelchair.

She had no recollection of the crash but from time to time asked me, "How did I end up here anyway?" Only when she was having a very good day, perhaps every couple of months, would she ask about him.

"Is my husband picking me up soon?"

I'd bluff an answer; her mind wouldn't be able to hang on to the question for long.

Despite being the most highly medicated resident on the unit, all the pills provided her with only short periods of relief. Her granddaughter told me Sally had been in a different nursing home before coming to us and that things were better here. Before, there had been seizures, something we had managed to get under control. It was hard to imagine her condition any worse. It seemed every nerve ending in her body was on fire. I'd watch her smiling face begin to contort and I knew what was coming. Her teeth would grind together and in her deep raspy voice the moaning would start: "Oh Grandma." "Oh Grandma." Her chanting would continue unabated until she received more medication. The pills would snuff things out for awhile, maybe an hour or two, but then a spark, a flicker, and the flames would return. There are limits to how much medication a person can have within a certain time frame. Watching helplessly as she tried desperately to escape her own body, her torment would tighten my grip and my stomach as well. The fire burned until the clock said it was all right to administer more medication. These weren't attacks; something that came over her from time to time. This was her life. Unbearable pain followed by short respites of relief, yet she never complained. During calm moments I asked many times about her Grandma. Had they been close? Were you raised by your Grandma? She never gave me an answer. It was as if she didn't understand the question.

She was not easy to be around when she was suffering. Loud, repetitive, like nails on a chalkboard, her cries put everyone on edge. Mother Teresa would have clenched her fists. Yet how could you not care?

Sometimes groups of official visitors arrived: County Board members, City Council members perhaps. They came in large groups, all dressed up, to look the place over. They never stayed on our unit very long. I know it's a big building with a lot to see.

But one minute? Maybe two? In all my time here, none of those visitors ever asked a question of me, or of any staff member I'm aware of. Not one of them ever went near a resident.

When Sally was being loud and difficult, most of these people couldn't even muster a glance in her direction.

I know if I were in the group I would tell the others, "Hey, I'm going to sit with this lady awhile. I'm gonna ask some questions, and try to learn a few things."

Instead, they walk through, hands in pockets or arms folded in front of them, smiling and nodding. Then, like ants hurrying for a smashed cantaloupe, this bunch of nervous looking, well-dressed people with good intentions I'm sure, make a beeline for the door.

Shouldn't there be more than a check in the mail? It just seems so impersonal. Maybe we are becoming desensitized because of the staggering numbers. By the year 2029, all baby boomers will have reached age 65. Predictions then estimate 615,000 new Alzheimer's and dementia cases a year. In 1960 there were 500,000 people in mental institutions in the entire country. But numbers are for Wall Street. Each of these people has a story worth reading.

They finally figured out some actual work for me to do, straightening and changing all the beds, and I started taking

Sally along to "help." It was spur of the moment. She was
being so loud, and I thought it would give everybody else a
break. It turned into a routine which lasted for years, and
the benefits were twofold. If she was having a hard time, I
wheeled her away from everyone else and kept her with me.
If she was okay, we talked about everything under the sun;
what I made for supper last night, how the fish were biting.
She spoke of having been in the Army and that she liked to
golf. What forever amazed me was that she could be such
a sweet, positive, warm person, given her circumstances.
Each morning I'd greet her in my best Brooklyn accent;
     "Yo, Sal. How you doin?"
     She'd smile and answer, "How are you doing?"
     "No no no. How *you* doin?"
     Again she'd answer, "How are you doing?"
     We sang her favorite song, "My Darling Clementine,"
and on walks down the hallways, she joined in as I taught
her "You Picked a Fine Time to Leave Me, Lucille." We were
awful singers, but made plans to take our talent on the road.
     If I heard her yelling in the afternoon while she was
lying down, I would sometimes go in, close the door and
sit with her. My job allowed me the freedom to go wherever
I thought I might do the most good. Much of our time
together, I simply sat holding her hand and bearing witness
to her suffering. There was no remedy.
     I wanted her to have the benefit of fresh air, but no matter
how nice the weather, despite sunglasses, a hat and a light
blanket, her system wouldn't tolerate it. After only a minute
she'd begin to tremble and ask to be taken back inside.
     It's fair to say that I spent more time with Sally than with
any other resident. She simply seemed to have the greatest
need. But I didn't always live up to my end of the bargain.
One morning she was with me while I changed the beds,
and she was having a rough time. My patience failed me.

"Sally, please. Stop yelling!"

Usually when she was loud and in the throes of pain, nothing could pull her out of it. This time, however, she did stop long enough to look at me and say, "You don't really love me."

Love was not a subject we had ever discussed. Certainly she wasn't mentioning love in the normal context one might assume in a man-woman relationship. She was questioning how much I cared. I knew we had grown close and that she liked and needed me. But love?

This book is of little value if it isn't truthful so I'll share a secret with you. There were times I prayed that Sally's pain would be taken from her and given to me. Nothing permanent, I didn't think I had the sand for that, but for awhile at least.

When you travel life's highway with someone you care about and that person is suffering, there is a toll you'll pay simply by being along for the ride. Maybe my noble gesture was born from the knowledge that it *couldn't* really happen. Sally hadn't asked a question. "You don't really love me." It was a statement. Wasn't it reasonable to assume that she did love me? My coming here had been about wanting to help, but I never realized that the process might lead me in this deep. Sally's relatives visited when they could but it was her caregivers who were Sally's family most of the time. Her son lived nearby, but was only able to visit in late evening, a time when Sally was usually asleep. She woke up to us, laughed with us and cried out to us. Like a helpless child, she was entrusted to us. Maybe that's why I prayed what I did. Ashamed of having lost my composure, I felt my shoulders go slack. I had failed someone who looked up to me above all others. When I knelt down that night I asked for forgiveness.

"Please help me do better tomorrow."

Over the years, I prayed those words often. When I was about to lose my patience and was able to stop myself, I knew He was tapping me on the shoulder. I was being reminded.

I'm not supposed to have it, but I've got a picture of Sally. I had it framed and it sits on my bedroom dresser. Looking at it makes me smile every time. If the rest of my life is of benefit to no one else, I know I did well by Sally. I will always remember my time with her and be grateful for it. Our relationship hasn't given me a completely clear conscience. But at least on judgment day when all my wrongs are being added up, I'll jump up and down and point to the one thing I think I got right.

A couple years after Sally's death I saw her granddaughter again. She came up to me teary-eyed, and thanked me for my efforts on her grandma's behalf. She didn't realize what Sally and I had together had nothing to do with the person I am. The good things all came from Sally, and the person she was. I have never met a braver heart.

On the night she died, I stayed after work for awhile to be with her. Eventually I left, but at 10:00 p.m., knowing I wouldn't be able to sleep, I went back to the nursing home. Her eyes were closed, her breathing labored. I prayed. I held her hand and talked. They say people can still hear you. I told her I loved her. Arriving for work the next morning, I went straight to her room. Her suffering was over. I never took anyone along to help me make beds again.

According to the Alzheimer's Foundation, at age sixty-five, one in eight people will show signs of dementia. By age eighty-five, that number grows to one in two.

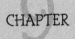

If that's Upper D, I'm Not Here

*U*pper D watches over a unique group of people. No two are alike, but all have characteristics that could be described as "unusual." Most are able to walk and talk. For reasons that vary with each individual they are unable to fend for themselves within the community. The nursing home is a safe haven.

Now and then Upper D would be short a staff member and would call our unit to see if I could help them out. My first experience with an Upper D resident came when I accompanied Big Clyde to a doctor appointment. Clyde's proportions could be compared to a mid-sized apartment building, which makes him appear a little intimidating. Getting Clyde up and sitting on the exam table took some doing. Next we had to get him prone. I gave a sigh of relief when that was accomplished. That's when he announced he needed to use the bathroom. The terrified female hospital staff didn't want any part of it and the chore landed in my squeamish lap. After several minutes of pushing and pulling I finally had him upright, only to discover he no-longer needed the bathroom. He was soaked. We hadn't brought extra clothes along. After a frantic search, one of the women handed me a goofy looking hospital gown, the largest she could find. It was barely big enough to cover the main parts for the ride home.

Peggy is another citizen of Upper D and someone you'd like. Sweets are her greatest love, but when we hand her a candy bar we're careful to keep our fingers out of the way. She rips the wrappers off with her teeth! We were walking down the hall one afternoon when she suddenly reached out and pulled a fire alarm.

"Peggy, don't do that!"

"I didn't do that."

"I saw you!"

"No you didn't."

At our musical events I slow danced with Peggy a time or two and was thrilled to finally discover a dance partner as utterly devoid of rhythm as I was. We didn't exactly glide across the dance floor, but stumbled and bumbled like a couple of flawed robots. Our individual dimensions were also a hindrance. Her eyes were perfectly level with my belly button. To anyone watching it must have looked like a bowling ball with feet being led around by an arthritic giraffe.

We got another call from Upper D. A new resident had arrived, somewhat unexpectedly, and there was no one to watch him. They asked me to come up and sit with him until they learned more about the guy and got all the paperwork in order. When I arrived he was relaxing in a lounge chair looking calm as an over-tired turtle while a nurse questioned him. I judged him to be about my age and was informed he had recently suffered a brain injury while working on his construction job. Her only instructions to me were, "Don't let him get up and walk around." No sooner had the nurse left when this guy flew out of his chair like a teenager after a ringing telephone. I grabbed him by the arm and pleaded, "Why don't we sit down Earl? Come on Earl, let's sit over here."

Earl had arms like a mountain gorilla and he dragged me around the unit like a chew toy. We visited every nook and cranny, every bedroom, every bathroom.

"See, see there" he would say, pointing at a bathroom wall.

Inquiring exactly what I was supposed to be looking at agitated Earl. I pictured a brawl inside a phone booth. Knowing such an occurrence would have a negative impact on my quality of life I decided to stop asking stupid questions.

Round and round the unit we went, like two mice in a giant maze, with Earl pointing out walls. Once I acknowledged that I saw the walls, away we'd go again. After three hours, someone came to relieve me. During our time together Earl and I never sat down for one cotton-pickin' minute. He seemed fine, I was exhausted. I never saw him again. There have been times since that day with Earl when I find myself standing in front of a wall. Just staring.

Upper D called again.

"Is there any way you could take one of our residents to a doctor appointment?"

What the heck, I like meeting new people. Janet was a little rough around the edges, but seemed okay. During the ride over she talked about her family and a laundry list of personal health problems. When it came time for her exam, I stayed behind to wait. A short time later I was told it was okay for me to go in and collect her. Janet and the doctor were exchanging small talk. Everyone was smiling, being cordial. I was relieved everything had gone well.

We said our goodbyes and were turning to leave when Janet, her voice suddenly turning to ice, faced the doctor and growled, "I'm going to sue you for every penny you've got!" The look on the doctor's face was priceless.

Back on Upper D I told some of the staff what had happened, and they all chimed in unison, "Yep, that's our Janet."

∽ ∾

We were having a party on our unit, and brought some of the residents from Upper D to join us. A thin, grizzled, smug-looking guy in a wheelchair was wheeled up to our piano. Pete sported a three-day beard and wore a baseball cap cocked to one side. The man looked like he'd been around the block a few times. His overall appearance suggested a lot of things but musical talent wasn't one of them.

No one expected much when he began playing but to everyone's surprise, he was really good. As the final song ended, we all smiled and applauded. I regretted forming an opinion about the man before even meeting him.

Then Pete turned in his chair and said, "Any of you don't like it can kiss my ass!"

To hear a performance personally, you'd have to come to the nursing home. Just follow the arrows to the elevator, press two for second floor, and it's the first locked door on your right.

∽ ⌒

I was on break outside having a smoke. Dave, a guy who had worked there for years, was with me. It was nice shooting the breeze with a man for a change. We had similarities in that we'd both been divorced. It was a subject we had discussed from time to time that I'd better not go into here. Around these parts there's a lawyer under every woodpile, twiddling his thumbs. Dave's got a big heart and loves the people he takes care of. He had worked with troubled youth before coming to the nursing home.

Near us, a large window allowed a view inside the building. When a figure walked past, Dave remarked, "There goes Big Johnny."

I'd seen the passerby many times around the building wearing a volunteer badge, usually pushing wheelchair residents to the beauty parlor or wherever. If you passed him in the hallway ten times in ten minutes, he would say "Good morning" to you every time. The guy was big all right, and always wore bib overalls.

"You know him?" I asked.

"Big Johnny? Sure I know him, used to be on Upper D."

"He worked there?"

"Hell no, he lived there!"

Dave leaned in; he had something to talk about.

"Big Johnny's a pussycat now," he told me, "but you should have seen him way back when." Dave lit another cigarette, shifting his weight. I had a feeling this was gonna be good.

"When Big Johnny's eyes got big, and he was kinda starin'," Dave began, already a little out of breath, "oh man, get ready! Back then, the nurse's station had one of those half doors. There was no top to it, and you could reach right in. One day I see Big Johnny headed for the nurse's station. He had that look in his eye, and there was nobody in there but the nurse. I hustle over and get between him and the nurse. He's starin' at me with those eyes, and he says he wants more medication. I tell him, 'No, it's not time yet.'

Next thing I know I'm in an ambulance, and this guy says, 'Don't try to talk. I think your jaw is broke!'"

Dave was smiling, shaking his head. "Yeah, I know Big Johnny. Those were the days. Not like now, with all the rules and stuff."

"We had this guy Oscar, a wild man, built like a tank. On bath day, six of us would grab a mattress and bullrush him."

Dave leaned back, deep in thought. The ash on his cigarette grew long. In the still air, smoke lingered above us like a fond memory. His eyes began to mist over. He had the look of a man recalling the birth of a first child. I would have loved to ask him more, but decided against it. Better to respect the moment.

Death from Alzheimer's disease usually occurs from an infection or a failure of other body systems.

CHAPTER 10

Bingo

The facility utilizes volunteers as much as possible. Most often they were women, and up there in age; one banana peel away from taking up residence themselves. There were lots of small, useful tasks they helped out with; serving coffee, reading aloud, or just visiting people. They usually wore sweatshirts with hearts, teddy bears, and *World's Best Grandma*, stitched somewhere on the front, a half box of Kleenex stuffed up one sleeve. Some wore chains around their necks like my mother did, with a house key hanging from it. When they'd get together with the residents, it was hard to tell who was who. We gave them badges to wear so there weren't any embarrassing mix-ups. For the most part, they worked on the nursing home end of the building, away from the dementia area.

We did have one lady helping us out. Her name was Stella and I assumed she was a volunteer. She only worked a few hours each week, and it turned out she drew a small wage. That was good news to me, as it meant I was no longer at the bottom of the monetary food chain. Stella was quite spry, so it surprised me a little when she mentioned she had recently turned eighty.

A little help is always appreciated, but she had one habit that had me grinding my teeth. The act of taking someone in a wheelchair off the unit requires you to push the door open with one hand, while pushing the wheelchair with the other. Stretching and a certain amount of strength were required. Stella found this difficult, and took to going out backwards, pushing the door open with her butt, and leaving both hands free to pull the chair.

This was a reasonable solution and one that I'd utilized myself on occasion. But here's what got me. If I happened to see Stella pushing someone, headed for the door, I'd run over and hold it open for her. She backed out anyway!

That does not make sense. The door is open! Just walk out for crying out loud!

"Thank you, Chuck," she'd say, backing her way past me.

From time to time, I helped out with Bingo at the nursing home. It's a lot different from the game that is played on the dementia wards. Obviously, folks on our units needed a lot of help, not only with playing the game, but with picking a prize. Nobody went home without a prize. Trying to eat the bingo chips was a reality we dealt with often, but there was no such problem at the nursing home. There, players played their own cards and picked their own prizes. Each game took about a month. Why so long?

Everyone was deaf. Each called number had to be repeated at a full yell several hundred times. Slowly.

I was usually in charge of passing out the prizes. We spread them out on a large tray from which the winner could select one. Prizes ranged from drinks and snacks to picture frames, small albums, stuffed toys and jewelry. The jewelry always went first. These ladies loved jewelry, but deciding could be so difficult. The gold butterfly pin or the Eiffel Tower earrings?

"Gertie, what do you think?"

"What?"

"Which should I pick?"

"Pick what?"

"Can you help me pick a prize?"

"What's wrong with your eyes?"

Meanwhile, fifty people behind me would be yelling BINGO! I'd start to lose it.

"Everything is silver, I was looking for something in green."

"Wait a week, it'll be green."

When a tray was nearly empty, we restocked it. Then past winners wanted to look at the new tray, interested now in a merchandise exchange.

"Gertie, should I trade the butterfly pin for the Panda necklace?"

"What?"

"Should I choose the necklace, or the pin?"

"Who committed a sin?!"

From time to time, we played a version of Bingo called Blackout. Rather than needing five numbers in a row, a player's entire card needed to be filled before a winner was called. Invariably, five numbers in, someone yelled "Bingo!" Then of course, we needed to explain about the new game again, that the entire card needed to be filled. If there were one hundred people playing, this explanation would need to be repeated one hundred times.

Like I said, about a month.

Every now and then, I would take all the jewelry off the tray, fill my fingers with rings, and wrap dozen's of necklaces around my neck. Then I'd walk around and say, "Sorry, we're all out of jewelry."

Some would hesitate a moment, then laugh, but others didn't see the humor. Whether it was something from the Dollar Store or the Hope Diamond, you didn't mess around with these women and their jewelry.

୭ ௧

There's an atrium on the second floor where I often took dementia residents with the hope they might enjoy watching the birds. I was surprised to learn that someone who I was certain would find enjoyment there had no interest at all. By the same token, someone like Mabel, who was forever fussing and fuming, found great delight in the experience. Attention span and the ability to recognize play key roles during activities with dementia patients. We included everyone, regardless of what we thought their capabilities might be.

On one occasion, while a resident and I were visiting the atrium, I noticed a lady sitting in her wheelchair crying. I asked what was wrong.

"It hasn't been a good day," she explained.

She'd received news that both of her daughters were very ill. I tried my best to console her but didn't make much headway. Eventually I had to leave, and the incident put a damper on my day as well.

Before work the next morning, I stopped at a gas station and bought a couple of roses, thinking I could drop them off and hopefully, cheer her up. Once on her floor, I couldn't find her. I tried to describe her to the unit nurse, but not knowing the woman's name left us both frustrated. A wheelchair and grey hair weren't the most helpful clues in those surroundings. When I mentioned that she had two daughters and they were ill, the nurse laughed.

"Oh, you mean Thelma! She's been moved to a dementia unit."

I punched in and there sat Thelma, happy as a chipmunk on a peanut ranch. I went over, introduced myself, and gave her the flowers. One of her daughters happened to be visiting and looked a little concerned about my motive. Eventually she thanked me for the gesture.

About 10% of Americans who suffer from Alzheimer's are under the age of 65.

CHAPTER 11

Friends of Mine

Nursing assistants work a lot of overtime. For many it's a financial necessity. I've always been amazed that someone taking care of a person's seriously ill Mom or Dad would probably do better hawking bananas at Kwik Trip. It shouldn't be a red flag that nursing home employees are under qualified. The ones who danced in there thinking it would be an eight maids-a-milking setting were either quickly disillusioned or weeded out. Although a few guys are sprinkled in here and there, the nursing assistant position is dominated by females. The work is hard, the hours are long, with difficulties unimaginable to someone not in the know. Yet they duck, they dodge, sometimes they take direct hits, and still they remain. They stay for the residents as much as for the paycheck. Many of them are young, just getting started in life and scrambling to make ends meet. Their dedication is, in my opinion, a testament to the goodness in people and showcases how much they care.

My situation was a little different. I came here at a time in my life when money was not as big a concern. It was also the point in my life where I had arrived at the "cliff's edge" mentioned at the beginning of this book on the Author's Note page. Driving a delivery truck is hard work. If the company you work for is United Parcel Service, its hard work times three. Company expectations are, dare I say, unreasonable. The pace, icy roads and walkways, packages that keep getting bigger and heavier. The weight limit has grown to one hundred and fifty pounds per box, and loading docks that are fine for a semi driver leave a UPS man staring upwards with hundreds, if not thousands of pounds to unload. Over the years I'd taken a lot of nasty falls on the ice and seriously strained my back more times than I can count. I once stepped into someone's pitch black garage and immediately tumbled down eleven concrete steps. I know there were eleven. I counted them when I came to.

Twice, fellow motorists tried to kill me. The first was a young woman in an old station wagon with no brakes, coming down a steep hill. She would later tell the officer, "I didn't know what to do, so I put it in neutral and closed my eyes." *That's a plan?* She hit me broadside, sending me across three lanes of traffic and through a cyclone fence. My truck came to a stop inches from a large sign that read "WELCOME TO MARATHON PARK." She would later argue the damage done to my truck was not her fault; it was the damn fence that caused all the havoc. Once I'd come to a stop, I sat dazed for a second, then opened the door, thinking I would get out. Feeling a bit woozy, I settled back in as an elderly man walked by. After staring at me for the longest time in silence, he finally thought of something worth commenting about.

"Yeah, yer head's bleeding."

The second attempt involved a twenty-one year old man driving drunk. We were on the highway and police estimated his speed at ninety to one hundred miles an hour when he rear-ended me. It was near the end of the day and my smaller truck was about empty. The impact forced me off the road and my truck rolled once, twice, or three times, depending on which witness account you want to believe. Personally, I was too busy applying a death grip to the steering wheel to count. The truck then flipped end over end before coming to rest on its side. I was stuck inside, unable to move, and very conscious of the strong odor of gasoline. It was rush hour, and traffic was backed up far behind the accident scene. A semi-driver and fellow Teamster, eventually came over, undid my seatbelt, and pulled me through the opening where the windshield had just been. When I was freed, I turned a fearful eye back down the highway, still unsure of what had struck me. One hundred yards away a pick-up truck rested on its side. The truck's driver lay face down in the road. I implored God to spare his life. We were taken to the hospital in separate ambulances and as I was being prepared for a CAT scan, a policeman arrived to interview me. I learned not only had the other driver been drinking, but he was still intoxicated and being combative. Now I wanted God to keep him alive until I could get my hands on him.

I had injuries to an elbow and shoulder which meant months of excruciating physical therapy and a finger badly broken in two places. After this second crash I spent a year in counseling, where an expert worked to erase the fear I experienced getting behind the wheel each morning.

My last couple of years at UPS, I would drive back to the terminal at night dreaming about the day I could hang it up, but was always left wondering, "what then?" Maggie suggested a school bus driver. After having raised four kids, my only response was, "You've got to be kidding."

"Maybe I'll open a little restaurant. I make really good hard boiled eggs." I was lost, until the situation with mother began to unfold. North Central Health Care offered intangible rewards UPS couldn't. Instead of fifty or more hours a week I could work thirty-two. Not an overload, but enough to keep me out of trouble. At UPS I was always on the run. I met many people, but got to know very few. The nursing home dementia units are the opposite. A core group of people I would get to know intimately. People like Noreen.

~∽ ⌒∽

You've got to play the hand you're dealt, an expression heard all the time. It was probably coined by someone holding a royal flush.

In the game of life, Noreen occupied a cold seat when the cards were passed. She did not have dementia; she never got far enough to qualify. Bi-polar and learning disabled only begin to describe her many obstacles. I stood with the charge nurse when Noreen approached, apparently upset. Looking the nurse in the eye she didn't mince words.

"I'm going to kill you." She followed that by pointing to the floor and casually remarking, "I like your shoes." Noreen's in her mid-sixties, she looks like she's in her forties, even with no teeth, and acts like she's three.

People like Noreen often appear younger than their age. They haven't had to worry about a mortgage payment, raising kids, or holding down a job. The goal every day is to wake up. Anything after that is gravy.

Her childish behavior could be problematic. I guessed her weight to be pushing two hundred pounds. Thinking she had fallen, staff came running when they saw Noreen sprawled on the floor. They forgot that when she didn't want to do something she'd simply drop to the floor and refuse to budge. Hand her a crayon, and in a few minutes the entire unit needed repainting. Paper was for tearing into thousands of pieces. If it takes an entire village to raise a child, that's pretty much what we had going on there.

Noreen had been on the unit for years and despite her shenanigans, she was as loveable as a puppy. The office staff was particularly fond of her, probably because they weren't the ones cleaning up her messes. She had an appetite that rivaled anything in the animal kingdom, willing to eat anything that didn't move. On second thought, willing to eat *anything*. Table manners? There weren't any. After eating, she appeared to have been in a food fight. We didn't bring a washcloth to clean her up. We brought a mop, bucket and as many bath towels as possible.

Every year around Christmas a dance is held in downtown Wausau for the learning disabled. With no male escort Noreen had never attended. Then someone with way too much time on their hands realized the unit had someone available to fill the role. I was skeptical. If I'd ever entertained fantasies of a dream date, this wasn't it.

All the women made a fuss getting Noreen ready for her big night out. A desperate search for the perfect dress, getting her hair styled, nails painted, lipstick applied. The million and one things a woman needed to do before she could walk out the door. The nursing home provided a car for our use. The vehicle was on the small side, and Noreen was a long way from being steady on her feet. Coordination was non-existent. Petite was left behind thousands of donuts ago. The difficulty getting her properly positioned in the front seat, belt secured, was akin to putting a man on the moon. Did I mention I have back problems?

Over the years, Noreen and I attended several dances and I must say, I was happily surprised and impressed. Though the locations varied, the surroundings were always first rate. Free soft drinks and snacks the entire night, and a DJ who gave every effort to make the evening the "real deal" for individuals whose lives revolved around rules and regimen. Dance partners came in all shapes and sizes, with prejudice towards no one. The window to innocence was flung open, and childlike hearts danced not just to music, but to the joy of opportunity. Dreams of tomorrow are born on nights like these.

The first couple years Noreen and I danced quite a bit. I'm not sure there's a name for the style we had. Facing each other several feet apart, we stretched out til we could clasp hands and swing our arms from side to side. I was grateful there wasn't any footwork involved. To repeat, rhythm is not one of my strong points. After that first year or two, stamina became an issue. We were both getting older. The snack table became our hangout.

Noreen's overall health had always been a concern and slowly began to worsen. It got to the point where a feeding tube had to be inserted. Food, the one thing in this world that gave her true enjoyment, had literally been taken off the table. With the feeding tube, her condition seemed to stabilize, but not to the point where she was the same old Noreen. Something was amiss.

Noreen was eventually moved from our unit to Upper D. I'm sure there were relevant reasons why that took place but personally, I could never figure it out. She'd been with us so long. Shortly after her move, and perhaps in retaliation for it, she was up to her old tricks again, jamming towels into her toilet and flooding Upper D.

Word spread quickly when she began to fail, and I went up to pay her a visit. She was in bed, asleep, and it was obvious that her time was getting close. I said a few prayers. And as Dad had taught me a gentleman is obliged to do, I thanked her for the dance.

As I work to fill these pages it's apparent to me the many good times, the laughs, or the instances when something dreadfully unexpected happened, are easy to bring to mind and write about. It's the *moments* that are harder to recall. The times where I was forced to stop for a second in mid-stream to say, "Thank you, Jesus." The hundreds of occasions when someone reached for my hand, as if it were the only thing in the world that mattered. When I watched someone, a person whose thought process had been destroyed, attempting to pray. The time Eileen, her vocabulary by then so limited, smiled at me.

"You're good," she said. High praise considering it came from someone who seldom spoke. I knew what she was trying to say, and it meant so much. What else can someone in Eileen's situation give you in return for your efforts? Moments. How is it they lack the capacity to fill a book, yet, can fill a life?

One special moment I experienced demonstrates how important it is to include everyone and never take anything for granted. While the learning disabled have a holiday dance downtown, each December our unit put on a Christmas party for residents and their families. Despite all of the work it's an event the staff enjoys. The facility supplies musical entertainment, snacks, drinks, and special desserts. The CNAs put extra effort into making sure each resident looks their best. The women have their hair done and the men wear dress shirts and ties. While the rest of the staff wears reindeer or elf hats, I suffer a slow, hot death underneath a Santa Claus suit, fake beard and winter boots. When she can, Maggie stops by to help out. And that makes the day special for me. We dance, make our way from one table to the next, making sure we visit with everyone. Seeing these people smiling, laughing, having a good time, brings so much satisfaction you want to squeeze out every last drop.

The party was nearly over and people began to leave as I made my way around the crowd for the second or third time. I noticed Francis sitting alone, his family had apparently left. Francis was a husband, father, veteran, pilot and tree farmer. Now he has Alzheimer's. Unable to walk, talk, or express himself in any way. Other than sitting near a group where something is going on, he takes part in no activities. While I wouldn't describe his face as expressionless, it was always difficult to decipher what he thought or felt. There were times when he seemed to be smiling, but it wasn't something I welcomed, the expression could appear somehow sinister. I'd been jumping and jingling, doing my best Saint Nick impressions, when I knelt down and patted him on the knee.

"Merry Christmas, Francis. I hope you and your family had a good time."

His body had not yet forgotten how to cry. With that awkward smile across his lips, tears trickling down his cheeks, Francis took hold of my wrist, raised my arm, and kissed the back of my hand. Sometimes, all the hours and days in a lifetime seem of little value when compared to one special moment.

◔◞ ◟◔

Getting to know the residents, I slowly discovered my favorites, so it's only natural there be someone at the other end of the spectrum. *Outcast* seemed a little strong, so what then? *Unfavorite?*

I am not suggesting she was ignored. Her needs were met with the same degree of care as everyone's. In fact, ignoring this woman was impossible. Using the palms of her hands, Frieda liked to pound on table tops. It could sound like a war going on and was bothersome to staff and residents alike. No admonishments from staff or threats from other residents did any good. She was oblivious. She just pounded away, staring at you wide-eyed, a huge toothless smile across her face. Or not toothless, depending on what she'd done with her dentures. We discovered them all over the place. It could be unnerving when you unknowingly sat down on a set of dentures. Frieda learned how to rotate them, top to bottom, bottom to top, without the use of her hands. Don't ask me how she did it. It was a gift.

When she pounded, I came running with pen and paper, an effort to redirect. Frieda was once a school teacher so I'd write down a sentence for her to copy: "*I leave my entire estate to Chuck.*" The penmanship was legible until she got to my name.

When the mood struck, she went from room to room, lying down in other people's beds that I had just made!

During meal time, residents wore clothing protectors, the professional description of a bib. Frieda knew where they were stored and visited the area frequently. She'd gather up an armload, roll each into a ball, then stuff them between the cushions of furniture around the Unit. We gathered them up and sent them back to laundry for re-washing. Fortunately, she only did this *constantly!*

Meal trays were wheeled in on a large cart. Protruding from each tray was a menu bearing the name of the person the tray was for, and a list of foods supplied for that specific individual. This was vital information when you consider residents with diabetes, weight control needs, swallowing issues, and so on.

Frieda made a game of this too, rushing to the cart and pulling out as many menu slips as possible before we could get to her. We wouldn't know whose tray was whose! Frieda's eating habits I won't even discuss. I'll just say it would've been nice if she'd made up her mind what to do with her teeth.

A nurse told me once that Frieda's constant grinning was a result of her medication. When she was up to her irritating antics that smile became a dagger. It had to be her father who penned the phrase, "*Wipe that smile off your face!*" But the smile was there, it was staying there, so it was in a person's best interest to get used to it. She no longer spoke but had a sizeable repertoire of yells and screeches she enjoyed sharing. There was an occasion when I thought I heard her say, "Philadelphia!" But who knows? I asked her politely several times to repeat herself, but she just ignored me. So-o-o, I had a hard time warming up to her, but people grow on you. That darn smile wore me down.

When it comes to lifestyles, even life styles with dementia, Frieda walked her own trail, going about her business each day unflappable, secure in the knowledge that the rest of the world was acting odd. I admired that.

I took nearly all of my residents on many walks, but never Frieda. The possibility never really crossed my mind. She walked well on her own, but some of her antics, even there, turned more than a few heads. One day, my sense of adventure apparently got the best of me and we strolled out the door, hand in hand. As we passed my bosses' office, the door was open. When she noticed who I had with me, she looked like a woman with an aspirin lodged in her throat.

We made our way from the behavior end of the building and set our course for the calmer confines of the nursing home. It was quiet there. People sat, visited, read the paper, and had coffee. I was just getting comfortable with my decision to take Frieda for a walk when she let loose an ear popping, blood curdling shriek, the likes of which Hollywood would find difficulty reproducing. Dozens of horrified faces turned our way. Staring back was a wide-eyed, toothless or not toothless, I don't remember, lady, with a huge grin on her face. I knew where there was one shriek there could be two. I quickened our pace, my mind desperate for a way to redirect.

I began to whistle softly. Nothing special, just whatever I could muster. I was relieved when Frieda took notice. What was I thinking? She, too, began to whistle but with an apparent need to out-do me. The pitch continued to grow until she was emitting a sound no reasonable person would identify as whistling. Once she reached her whistling limits, Frieda abandoned that effort and began blowing as hard as she could until she produced a sound of jet engine proportions. The hallway became a wind tunnel. We took our walks outside after that day.

A framed picture hung on the wall in Frieda's room. In it she's standing with a group of nice looking people in front of a church. A wedding perhaps? I wondered why she never got visitors. She approached the picture at times and scratched the glass with her fingernails. She did not do this with any other pictures or objects. I have to believe that she was somehow, in her own way, trying to reconnect with people she once knew, a life she once lived.

She did get a visitor one day, a court-appointed legal guardian. We saw them, from time to time, sent by the Court to check on the person they'd been assigned. They'd sit down together and go over papers and discuss legal matters, knowing full well their client hadn't a clue who they were, or what they were talking about. It was all legal formality. Even so, I'd always seen it done professionally.

Frieda's representative was a woman, and she was a looker. Short blond hair, stylish, a form fitting dress that ended just above the knee, and high heels. A woman who could turn a man's head. My neck is still a little sore. She explained to Frieda who she was and why she was visiting. She seemed nervous. Across from her, a smiling lady was rotating her teeth. The representative began reading hurriedly from a legal document, just as the pounding started. That was all it took.

"This is a waste of my time," she quickly muttered, and her high heels clicked their way to the door. Her entire manner seemed to say, "You and I both know I'm above all this."

Whenever I took one of my resident's to a doctor's appointment, or any occasion where we were out in public, I was always very defensive on their behalf. A *what-are-you-starin'-at* type of thing. This was an occasion like that. The beauty here was most assuredly skin deep. Like a supermarket tomato, the woman looked good, but she wasn't the real deal. As she was leaving, I wanted to say, *"Don't let the door hit you in the ass,"* but I was too busy staring.

I turned my attention back to Frieda, but she was no longer at the table. I found her lying down in someone else's room.

"Frieda! I just made that bed! AND STOP SMILING AT ME LIKE THAT!!"

❧ ❧

Violet wandered a lot. Many times she'd approach someone and just stand there beside them.

Often she searched for a bathroom. I found her one day in the kitchen. She had just pooped on the floor in front of the refrigerator. Personally, I thought the stove area seemed cozier. But Violet chose the frig. Why I don't know, you'd have to ask her.

Violet hailed from the northwest corner of the Badger state. She was barely five feet tall and at one time owned a restaurant. She won an award on the Unit for "Most Creative Sandwich," something that I believe had to do with chili and crackers. Oh, and pears. She could talk but seldom did, a rare quality in a woman. She had another way of expressing herself. Whatever we would address her about, she'd lower her chin to her chest, then look up at us with wide, innocent, puppy dog eyes. It'd get us every time.

Often she walked around looking for someone to comfort. Without a word, she'd simply place her hand on a shoulder and smile. If someone was seated with a blanket over them, Violet took great care to make sure the blanket covered properly. With her heart and probably some egg yolk on her sleeve she went about trying to help.

I do recall one occasion where she showed a bit of a stubborn streak. She walked right out the Unit door and into the hallway. An alarm immediately sounded. When I went to fetch her she wouldn't budge. It was clear she was on a mission somewhere down the hall. I could either come along or get out of the way. I went along (I do the same thing with my wife all the time). It was late afternoon, sundown syndrome time. Most office staff had already left for the day. We were near the end of the hall when we found an office door open and a secretary still inside typing. Violet turned to go in. This was apparently the place we'd been looking for. The secretary turned to us with a puzzled look, asking if there was something she could help us with.

"I would like to see the Principal," Violet stated.

There was some hesitation before the secretary figured out what was going on, but once she did she handled it perfectly. She informed Violet that the Principal had left for the day but would be back in the morning. With that, Violet was satisfied and we returned home.

I went with her to an eye appointment that turned out to be rather interesting. I wasn't worried about any problems. Violet was very docile and always tried her best to follow instructions. Though she wore eyeglasses when she first came to live with us, we had no vision records, therefore no way of knowing how good or bad Violet's eyesight was. Hence, the appointment. An assistant was giving this routine exam, but struggling. With Violet seated on one side of the room, she pointed to an eye chart on the opposite. It was a standard chart bearing letters, largest on top, getting smaller as you worked your way down. She urged her patient for quite some time to read a letter, any letter, but was getting no response, just the puppy-dog look.

She left the room to look for help, and returned shortly with the good doctor in tow. His demeanor made it clear he meant business, with no time for nonsense. Yanking the chart off the wall he put up a replacement, this one bearing pictures rather than letters. The first picture was the palm of a person's hand, with fingers spread wide. Pointing at the chart it sounded almost like a command.

"Tell me what you see here Violet."

Much to my surprise, Violet suddenly found her voice.

"A willow."

"A what?"

"A willow."

"A willow?!"

Grasping his right wrist with his other hand, he spread his fingers wide.

"The hand! Can't you see the HAND?"

His booming, impatient voice bounced off the walls of the small room. It was clear this guy was ill-equipped, and I didn't like him. Violet, however, was not intimidated.

Smiling back she replied, "I see a hand, holding a willow."

As far as I knew we still weren't sure how good or bad Violet's vision was, but she wasn't bumping into things.

Violet's husband was, by then, living in the nursing home. While his mind was sound, his body had discovered limitations. Most days he'd wheel himself down to spend time with her. Violet didn't really talk anymore. She might surprise you with a short sentence once a month, which would leave you wondering, "*Where did that come from?*" Her husband would lead her off to sit in a corner somewhere, holding her hand, until something caught her eye. Then she'd get up and walk away, leaving him to sit alone. Violet didn't know who he was.

∽ ∾

We had two other residents with marriage partners at the nursing home. One of the partners, a husband, was lucky. His wife remembered him. In fact, she constantly questioned his whereabouts. He visited daily, cuddling with her on the couch. It brought her peace and the chance for a nap. The remainder of the day she was moody and restless.

With the third couple, it was the husband who had dementia. His wife, whose health was marginal, came to see him as often as she could, usually a few times a week. While her husband still talked, there was no sense to the conversations. His answers bore no relevance to the questions she asked. She desperately sought his companionship, but any time spent with her seemed to be more out of obedience and following instructions, "Sit right here," than any recognition that this woman was his wife. At a staff softball game put on for the residents, I was forced to stop my umpire duties to go collect him. He'd deserted her in her wheelchair and was wandering aimlessly.

For about a year I volunteered with a faith-based organization in town. People who sign up are asked to lend a hand wherever they feel most qualified. It may be building wheelchair ramps or running errands. I suggested that I could supply a little respite to an individual caring for someone with dementia in their home. Since I worked four days a week, I felt comfortable that I'd have the time and energy to help a family. Before I could turn around I was up to four families, and it got to be too much. I insisted to the program's director that I couldn't possibly help with more than three families. Then she told me about an aging wife, so desperate for a break she paid $75 for a six-hour bus tour, and nearly $400 for a nurse to watch her husband while she was gone. With four families it seemed my phone was always ringing, and how do you say no to a little old lady who's wondering if it might be possible to slip out a short while to attend church?

I'm not at liberty to go into any detail regarding the families I helped while volunteering, but I will say that in one household the situation had reached the breaking point. An elderly wife with few resources was caring for her husband whose dementia, in my opinion, was already in the latter stages. It was a situation she had dealt with for many years, robbing her of a life of her own. Finally, in desperation, she reached out to her Pastor, who put her in touch with the volunteer organization. My experience reinforced what I already suspected. There's a great deal of need, hiding behind closed doors and drawn curtains. Aging partners are burdened with circumstances spinning more and more out of control. Adult children, often living out of town, sometimes out of state, are left to wonder and worry.

The effects of Alzheimer's reach far beyond those living with the disease. Caregiving at home for a loved one with Alzheimer's is more than difficult. Without a tremendous amount of help, the situation will eventually become overwhelming. From banking and legal affairs to toileting, the loved one will become totally dependent, a 24/7 proposition. Caregivers face physical and emotional exhaustion.

One of the female residents on our unit was the epitome of what you might picture a mother and grandmother to be. Despite overwhelming disabilities, "amazing grace" was still the description I used for her. Her children told me how hard it was for their dad to bring Mom here.

"She took care of me all these years," he'd say "and now, when she needs me…"

Augusta was a lady of large proportions. A power lift was needed to get her in and out of bed, the wheelchair, or on and off the toilet. Occasionally when in bed and needing cares, I was asked to come in and lend a hand rolling her on her side.

She was happy and jovial, with no clue as to her circumstance or surroundings. She'd been there for years, yet couldn't remember the staff from one day to the next. Her short-term memory was gone. Except when it came to me. Somehow she remembered me and would greet me by name. It was a phenomenon I can't explain. I didn't interact with her any more than with anyone else. She had a big, gushing smile and would greet me.

"Hiya Chuck!"

The rest of the staff would glare at me and ask, "How'd you get her to do that?"

I couldn't explain it then and I still can't.

The Hippocampus is the part of the brain controlling memory, and the first area attacked by Alzheimer's. Augusta loved music and could sing the words to every old song ever written. Yet you could pick up the dirty dishes in front of her, and she would want to know, "When are we going to eat?" If you explained that she'd just finished eating, Augusta would gush at you and laugh. That something might be wrong never occurred to her.

The best description I've ever heard regarding this type of short-term memory loss is to think of the brain as a tape recorder. The recorder takes in new information and files it away. Then one day it stops working. All the old information is still in the file, but anything new is denied entrance. The degree of damage can vary from person to person. In Augusta's case the loss was complete.

I never considered her memory problems to be something that would affect me, until I accompanied Augusta to a doctor's appointment. We were led into an exam room and asked to wait. A winter day, outside a heavy snowfall was coming down. A window in the room provided a view. A diagram of the human brain hung on the opposite wall. Augusta's neck was weak, causing her head to bobble whenever she turned it. She spied the picture on the wall and exclaimed, "Oh my God! A human brain!"

Her head then bobbled in the direction of the window, and she needed to tell me about another discovery.

"Oh my God! Look at it snow!"

Then back to the picture.

"Oh my God! A human brain!"

Back and forth, back and forth. The longest twenty minutes of my life!

When I stand before my creator, if He wants to know how I spent my time on earth, I'm going to answer, "*Studying the human brain and watching it snow with Augusta.*"

෴ ෴

When a new resident arrived, there was apprehension about what to expect, what challenges you might be presented with.

When Jed was wheeled through the door, we were all soon put at ease. Talkative and amiable, he was easy to like. He was a farmer through and through, with a strong Polish heritage. Jed was high functioning for our unit, which is why after a couple of months his family collected him and took him back home. We were happy to see that because it's an event we didn't witness often.

That's not to say Jed wasn't mixed-up. Most of his time with us he spent playing solitaire, not realizing half the cards laid on the floor where he'd dropped them. Our social worker sat down with him the first morning to ask some questions. It was standard procedure with new residents to try and determine at what level a person's faculties performed.

"Jed, I'd like to ask you some questions. But first, I'm going to tell you three words I'd like you to remember. When I'm done with my questions, I want you to tell me what those three words were. Do you think you can do that for me Jed?"

Jed had a way of dragging out his words. When he answered "okay," it came out "o-o-o-k-k-kay."

"Jed, the three words I want you to remember are: chair, window, and door. Chair, window, door. Will you try to remember those words Jed?"

"O-o-o-k-k-kay."

She began her questioning.

"Where are you from? What's your wife's name? How many children do you have?"

Jed did well. Our social worker wondered if Jed's admittance should be approved. Then came the test.

"Jed, can you tell me the three words I asked you to remember?"

"O-o-o-k-k-kay," answered Jed with a confident smile. "I gotta remember, don't piss in the combine."

ᘒ ᘓ

I've concluded that families of those with Alzheimer's come in four distinct categories. The first group is the one we see the most. They laugh and visit as best they can, still enjoying the company of the person they love. The second group comes a little less often. Instead of laughter, they may be brought to tears. The third group sits mortified, frozen by their surroundings, nearly as helpless as the person they've come to visit.

To all of these people I say "Thank You."

The last group we don't see because they are never here. There are instances where these families simply do not exist, but too often the hard truth is that they are busy elsewhere.

Leona was someone whose sad, innocent face melted your heart. In her mid-nineties, she weighed less than 100 pounds, and subsisted on nibbles of food, vitamin drinks and the tea she so loved. Painfully fragile, Leona's days were spent asleep in bed. Staff members got her up an hour or so before each meal. Wrapped in blankets, her frail body forever sought warmth. As I talked with her, she told me that she was a secretary, currently working for a large firm in Milwaukee. But this wasn't what she really wanted to talk about. What mattered to Leona most was that I knew she had four children, Kyle, Danny, William and Sarah. I could question her about other things, change the subject, bring up current events, but I wouldn't get far. It was imperative I was aware she had four children, Kyle, Danny, William and Sarah. I had never met Kyle, Danny, William or Sarah. *Where on earth could they be, and what could possibly be more important to them than visiting their mother?* I bit my tongue til it bled. Exceedingly difficult, this effort not to judge others.

Alzheimer's and dementia triple health care costs for people over age sixty-five.

CHAPTER 12

Nobody's Perfect

Each quarter all the CNA's were required to take a test. A little refresher course really. The entire process lasted only ten or fifteen minutes. More often than not it had to do with personal cares and my old friend, the dummy. Just knowing the testing was coming up filled me with dread. I'd try to explain that I didn't do personal cares, that it was not part of my job description, but those in charge insisted since I had the license, I needed to be included.

"What if there's an emergency?"

"What if a large number of residents come down with diarrhea and your co-workers are all home ill?"

"What if you're the only one available?"

I pointed out that in a situation like that I would go ahead and shoot myself, but to no avail. There seemed to be a perverse need to see me humiliated. Long ago I

figured out that in a diarrhea emergency it would be my job
to faint, or at the very least, get out of the way.

The testing was done in pairs. We needed to fill our
name in one of the available time slots. Whenever possible
I tried to sign up with someone I knew, someone who might
be sympathetic to my admitted incompetence. I'd let him or
her answer all the questions that are asked of us, then watch
intently as they stepped up to the dummy and performed
the required tasks correctly.

When it was my turn, I'd immediately labor to breathe,
my face flushed. My mind would go blank and I'd start
feeling faint. Holding my breath, I'd pick up a washcloth,
apply soap, extend my hand, and the nurse was already
screaming, "*Not that way!*"

After nearly five years of employment I was asked to work
on C Unit. It was twice the size of E Unit with double the
population. The nurse's station sat directly in the middle of
the huge room, effectively creating two distinct sides.

My move had to do with changes being made to more
effectively serve the residents. In the past, a patient was
admitted wherever space was available. The new concept was
aimed at each Unit, E and C, sides one and two, being more
specific to the different stages of dementia. The change
allowed people at the same stages to be housed together.

My former E Unit became home to people in the final
or near final stage, with activities designed more towards
sensory. It was suggested that whatever skills I had were
better suited to people in the earlier and mid- stages.
Leaving my old unit and so many memories behind was

difficult, but things had changed. The move was absolutely the right thing for me to do.

The nursing home hadn't escaped the economic downturn. There was speculation the place would be forced to close its doors. In an effort to re-vitalize, a new management team was brought in. The changes were immediate and ongoing.

Fiscal responsibility came first and as that was brought under control, all attention turned towards the residents and how they could be better served. Creation of units with the "stages" concept was one step.

Initiatives were geared to quality of life. A more home-like environment was created, a cultural change away from the traditional nursing home setting. The activity staff was expanded with more resources made available. Fireplaces were installed on each Unit. Even unit names were changed. Gone were E, C, and Upper D. People were welcomed to *Garden Side Crossing, Lake View Heights* and *Evergreen Place.* The number of residents per unit was reduced, creating more room, while allowing more time and attention for those who were there.

Clothing protectors were discarded and replaced with cloth napkins. New food machines arrived, replacing the old meal carts. The machines produced heat, keeping food warm until a person was ready to eat. People could sleep in if they wanted to. No more, "It's time to get up." Plans were underway to adopt street names for the hallways, possibly even residents' rooms. Instead of Room E103, a sign above the door might proclaim that this is "Janet's House." I'd also heard rumors about allowing pets.

I knew some of the residents at my new assignment, *Garden Side Crossing,* but there was an equal number I had yet to meet. One of the ladies I became acquainted with was a joy to be around, until I'd get her to the dinner table. I would beg, plead, cajole, but nothing I tried could get her to open her mouth. I was completely frustrated, until a co-worker noticed my plight and took me aside. Her advice was to stop being so polite, stop asking the lady if she would like a bite of food, just give it to her. I returned to my table and without saying a word, raised a spoon to the woman's lips. Low and behold, away we went! Getting to know the person you were caring for made all the difference, little things meant a lot. And it could, at times, be difficult.

One of the ladies came to us in her mid- fifties. Her dementia was already severe but was considered "early onset." Up to 10% of those with Alzheimer's are in their forties or fifties, classifying them as "early onset." In the U.S. that's about 400,000 people. She wandered, babbled on and on, and responded to no one except her husband, who traveled a considerable distance to visit her every couple of days. I'd never met her teenage children.

There is a Hmong population here in town, and while people from the Southeastern Asian culture tend to take care of their own, we had a couple individuals who came to live with us. Both were female. The first has passed on but will always be remembered as extremely outgoing with a sunny disposition that endeared her to everyone. She spoke no English, yet she'd babble constantly, insisting that you pay attention. She was forever giving me backrubs, but I assure you, they were not solicited. It got to the point that, seeing her coming, I'd cringe, swallow hard, and try to hide. She loved doing it, but the woman had hands like a bull rider. By the time she finished I'd have tears in my eyes. Cleaning her room and organizing her things after she had died, we discovered a treasure trove of eating utensils, crayons, pictures, and miscellaneous things from around the Unit that she had been hoarding for safe keeping.

The second woman had the same language barrier and suffered dementia too pronounced to establish much of a relationship. Serving her food, I'd set it down and run, never sure if it would be eaten or launched. The facility tried to provide food suited to her nationality but had limited success. She was seated alone during meal time because I wasn't kidding about food being launched. From time to time family members visited, bringing her food from home, and most times she'd do better with that.

One day she delivered a tirade aimed at me and I asked a Hmong co-worker exactly what was being said. Her answer was not printable. I'll just call it unflattering and leave it at that. With only gestures and, from time to time, eye contact as communication tools, and with dementia thrown into the mix, it's not hard to imagine the difficulty and frustration experienced when trying to help someone from an origin and culture different than your own.

Actually, there was an Asian male resident there at one time also. I never worked with him personally but I remember that he appeared young, possibly in his forties. That most certainly would classify him as Early Onset Alzheimer's. He was constantly on the move, refusing to sit down. His meals had to be served to him while he walked around and when he found displeasure with something he'd leg kick high in the air like an Asian fighter. It was in the staffs' best interest to stay to one side.

Richard, unable to feed himself, still managed to make a game out of meal time. Smiling at me, he would duck and dodge his head whenever I put a spoon to his lips. Meal times could be fun and relaxing. We never knew what conversation we might have with a person we were trying to feed. It could also be desperately frustrating when the pendulum swung the other way. Nothing brought me more anxiety or anguish than trying to help someone who could not, or would not, be fed. In most instances the men were easier to assist, had better appetites and were less picky. As dementia progressed nourishment often became an issue.

A man we lovingly referred to as Gramps would sometimes throw his food, and for reasons known only to him, began biting the end of his index finger to the point he'd actually gnawed the tip off. Gramps biting his finger demonstrates the power dementia can wield over those in its grasp.

Levity had a place on our dementia unit. At times it could be a god's send, but was never used to the extent it veiled awareness of what we were up against. Situations we faced made us laugh, cry, left us frustrated, or staring out the window utterly perplexed and searching for answers.

Not telling the truth, the laughter *and* the anguish, would be a disservice to those who struggle with Alzheimer's and related dementia, to this book, and to you, the reader. Getting Gramps to stop his destructive habit was not easily accomplished. I don't recall how the problem was eventually solved. I remember an oven mitt was put over the injured hand, then secured to his wrist with tape to prevent Gramps from pulling the mitt off. That effort had to be abandoned when federal regulations regarded what we were doing as a "restraint." That may sound ludicrous, but it was a reality staff members dealt with day in and day out, with every individual. Someone might be wandering, over-tired, acting out, or unsteady on their feet. We could lead them to a reclining chair in an effort to find them some comfort, but we were not allowed to put their feet up. This, too, would be considered a restraint.

Those who struggled the most at meal time were usually seated together. Problems arose such as "pocketing," storing food in the side of the mouth without swallowing. "Excessive chewing." A meal that should take minutes could turn into hours. Pureed foods and thickened liquids were often ordered, and therapists tried to work with an individual, but you can imagine the difficulty. Often, people simply refused to open their mouths. When it was an individual we had come to know and care about, while a tormented family watched their loved one decline, the helpless feeling that came over you was maddening.

The process repeated itself, day after day, meal after meal, until it reached a point where I recognized it as pure torment. I'd always tried to be a team player, going where help was needed without question. That being said, there were meal times when I surrendered, hurrying over to assist some of the guys. I simply could not endure the agony of what I was certain would turn out to be another exercise in futility, knowing that with each failure the eventual outcome inched closer.

∾ ∾

There are so many misconceptions about Alzheimer's patients. Almost always the culprit is lack of knowledge. A woman came to visit her mom, and while mom slept, we talked for the first time. She mentioned she was grateful.

"At least Mom's not mean."

When she repeated herself not a minute later I couldn't help myself.

"None of our people are mean," I told her. "They're just sick."

With that our conversation abruptly ended. I may have overstepped.

A man named Ed had recently been admitted. The female staff was leery of him, and not without reason. He could be aggressive. Sitting passively in a chair one moment, Ed could be on his feet and swinging the next. His anger it seemed, directed at whoever happened to be the closest. He had been at private nursing homes in the past, but things hadn't worked out. About six feet tall, of medium build, ruggedly handsome, he was a former logger from the Tomahawk area. His wife still lived in the home Ed had built himself. Twice while working, he had suffered head injuries from falling trees.

When I introduced myself to Ed, I told him that my family was from Tomahawk. Perhaps that stuck with him, explaining why we got along so well. His speech was affected, but listening closely, I could still pick up the gist of what he tried to say. Throughout the day we would shake hands often. Ours was a firm, confident, daughter-there's-someone-you-should-meet handshake. The kind of handshake men equal under the sun are supposed to have. No one could get a handle on what triggered Ed's anger, but I could shadow box with him, mess his hair, and he accepted it with a jovial spirit, like I'd been a trusted friend since grade school. The goodness in him was easy to recognize. The anger was the disease, not the man.

When I brought Ed a snack, he would break the cookie in two, wanting to share it with me. More than once I witnessed him holding a chair after he'd noticed a woman about to sit down. There was a bowling game I often set up for the residents. Everything was life- sized but made of plastic. A metal ramp was used, so no one had to actually roll the ball. I could never get Ed to play. All he ever wanted to do was help me pick up the fallen pins.

One day other aids came to me fussing that Ed had wandered into the wrong room, and was lying down in someone else's bed. The bed's owner was ill and needed to lie down, but Ed was having none of that, keeping everyone at bay. I suggested that everyone leave the room and give me a minute. Ed and I emerged from the room hand in hand a short time later.

"That's amazing," I heard someone say.

I led Ed to his room, took off his shoes and cap, and got him comfortable in his bed. He thanked me and apologized for the "mix-up."

Feeling pretty darn smug, I left the Unit for lunch at the cafeteria. It was pride before the fall. I opened the door just as a resident named Lettie was being wheeled in. Lettie's mood swings are in the nursing home's history books. One look in her eyes told me I was in the wrong place at the wrong time. In a wheelchair at the time, she was permitted the perfect angle. She took a good, hard swing, and landed her punch right at the spot Dad warned me about. Humbled in an instant, I folded up like a lawn chair. So much for smug.

Please don't think poorly of Lettie. Before she came to live with us, with no children or close relatives, she would ride the city buses, giving her money away to strangers. The manager of the apartment building where Lettie lived brought her to us. Had it not been for the kindness of that woman, God knows what Lettie's future might have been. She was a wonderful woman with a terrible disease. Writing about her in depth is something I won't attempt. Her issues are so complex I wouldn't know where to begin. I can tell you Lettie obsessed. A thought in her head would bother her throughout the day. Bother as in, "*My house just burned to the ground, boy that bothers me.*"

For one week I kept track of things that bothered Lettie.

Monday: She wanted me to return the money she loaned me. Throughout the day the amount varied, from several thousand dollars, to twenty-nine bucks and change.

Tuesday: The barking dog kept her up all night. Trying to explain the dog on the couch is a stuffed toy was not worth the effort.

Wednesday: She kept taking clothes out of other's rooms. She wanted to mail them to her niece for Christmas. It was February, and I wasn't sure she had a niece.

Thursday: She was mad at me for what I did to her leg yesterday.

"Don't pretend you don't remember!"

Friday: Why wasn't she invited to my wedding?

Saturday: She's never cooking for this many people again.

Sunday: My notes ended. No one was going to believe me anyway.

Lettie sometimes "zoned out" at the dinner table, staring off while her food got cold. She was completely capable of feeding herself, and would angrily insist, "I *am eating*" when questioned. She wouldn't let anyone help her, wouldn't let us take the food away, and long after everyone else's meal had ended, she might accept a little ice cream. She often refused to take her medication, so her love of ice cream was a tool the nurse used to get this task accomplished. Crushing Lettie's pills and inserting the results in a bowl of ice cream was often the only way. Researchers already know that a person's sense of taste, particularly our "sweet tooth," stays with us long after other senses have diminished. Programs are being conducted that might aid a dementia patient, by a learned process, to eventually associate medication with something sweet.

After a visit with relatives a resident showed Lettie the stuffed monkey she'd been given.

"Looks just like you," Lettie told her with a smile.

Whether it was sarcasm or a genuine attempt to be polite was anyone's guess. With Lettie you never knew.

ⵔⵔ ⵔⵔ

I was sitting with Ed one afternoon when his wife arrived for a visit. Seeing her approach, eyes that had grown dull and weary suddenly sparkled. He looked up at her and said one word.

"You."

Hand in hand she led him to his room. At the time I thought about what a sad thing I'd just witnessed. Now I recognize the beauty of that moment. She laid him down, and for a few hours a tired man found peace, safe in the warmth of the woman he now referred to as "you."

The annual prom dance was an occasion we always looked forward to and the last year of Ed's life he was voted Prom King. Dressed in a suit with white shirt and tie, Ed was undeniably handsome. He and his wife smiled as they posed for pictures. Large windows provided a perfect backdrop of Lake Wausau and Rib Mountain in the distance. It was a happy moment. But I could only smile and wish things could be different. I pictured a day when two people stood before witnesses and purchased each other's lives. No warranties or guarantees. But simply a vow that has led them to this time and place. To a last dance, and a love story nearing it's end. Coming to work at the nursing home, I never realized my presence could weave me so deeply into the fabric of other people's lives. At times I almost felt like an intruder.

Ed was a man I felt a kinship with and I liked him a lot. Had we known each other under different circumstances, I believe we could have been like brothers. His illness was aggressive and his stay was relatively short. The day before he died he still knew who I was, a glimpse of a smile crossed his face as he tried to acknowledge me. With so much taken from him, I found comfort knowing he left us safe in the knowledge that he still had one thing, a friend. If you do your best to keep people safe and offer them friendship, you've given them all you can, which is really all they are asking for.

Ed could relax now. There were no more falling trees above. Only a friendly sky.

$\sim$ $\sim$

The "lawn chair" episode with Lettie wasn't my only inglorious moment.

The use is more restricted now, but in the past, anyone deemed a "fall risk" sat on an alarm, a little pad that emitted a whistle when the person sitting on it tried to stand. Hearing the alarm, we'd hustle over and either assist the person with walking, or get them seated again.

I ran toward a sounding alarm when I tripped, fell, and slid right into the tub room. *Physician, heal thyself.*

I've been an innocent bystander in more than one food fight. Some of the guys liked to spit. At times their accuracy was amazing.

An unusual situation unfolded one morning with the arrival of two new residents, a mother and her son. They arrived accompanied by other family members, the entire group walking and talking, making it hard to decipher who was who. Our nurse and office staff was busy meeting and greeting these folks. I just went about my business, but at one point a lady from the group left the others and approached me. She wanted to know if I could let her out the door. Nodding her head towards the north, she stated she was interested in seeing the nursing home end of the building. She was polite and well-spoken and it seemed a reasonable request. I unlocked and held the door open for her. A few minutes later a receptionist stationed at the south end of the building called.

"I've got a woman here. She says she's looking for her son."

ᘒᘏ ᘒᘏ

The first thing you'd notice about Rose is her posture. I'd never seen her stand, but she was obviously a tall woman. She sat rigidly straight. Her rigidity was not due to stiffness or some quirk of dementia. I believe it had more to do with her upbringing.

Rose played our piano, and not too badly if you didn't mind the same song performed over and over. She had a beautiful smile and was nearly always pleasant, though late in the day she could get a little obstinate. Suddenly adventurous, she'd wheel herself into a room where someone was sleeping and inform her snoring discovery, "It's time to get up!"

Redirecting Rose was futile. She was on a mission from God. It occurs to me that I'd never seen anyone come to visit Rose. And, shame on me, I am clueless as to her family history. I'll chalk that up to Rose always being so amiable and seemingly content. Where the need was the greatest, you dug a little deeper, like the wheel that squeaked the loudest.

With Rose, "effort" never crossed my mind. I realize now that I've failed her. She was very easy to sit and talk to, and once she got hold of my hand I could expect to be there awhile. She enjoyed conversation, but her ability to articulate was diminished. Dementia had a serious impact on what must have been a pretty formidable vocabulary once upon a time.

Rolling through a sentence one second, her words suddenly twisted and tangled. Rose was happily unaware. Whatever she'd just asked me might as well have been in Greek. I didn't have the foggiest, but she was smiling, holding my hand, and wanting an answer.

Not knowing what to say, I'd usually come up with something.

"Um-m-m-m. How 'bout tomorrow?"

Recently, my neighbor's grandchild was baptized and my wife and I attended the occasion. Their church was new to me. I read the church bulletin and noticed a section that listed church members who were ill and needed remembering. There was Rose's name. I prayed extra hard.

ᜒ᠑ ᥉᠑

So often, family members saw the opportunity to unload, and expressed the extreme difficulties and gut wrenching emotions that accompanied having a loved one with Alzheimer's. There was no way for them to know that my mother was on C Unit, just down the hall.

Though I never took care of Mom professionally, I visited her during my breaks or after work. She became increasingly distant, often wheeling herself away from me after I'd sat down. To this day I don't know if it was Alzheimer's that made her act that way, or if she was angry with me for having placed her in a nursing home. Whichever the case, she was talking to me a lot less. Swallowing problems developed again, a circumstance she'd been hospitalized for in the past. It was odd that I was so at ease with the majority of people living there, yet I struggled with my own mother. Other residents I accepted at face value, but with Mother I wanted to turn the clock back. I made every effort to keep her close, as she drifted farther and farther away—with ears that no longer heard my voice.

While I was still assigned to E Unit, C Unit began serving more residents who needed feeding assistance. It was more than C Unit's staff could handle on their own, so I was required to go and assist them with the noon meal every day.

On one occasion, several tables were strung together, allowing enough room to accommodate ten or twelve people. Mother happened to be seated on one end. I was on the opposite end, assisting two people. At some point, I looked up to see Mother staring at me. She was smiling, in a moment of clarity perhaps, a look of pride on her face. Regarding the last months of my mother's life, it's the one moment I care to hang onto.

According to the Alzheimer's Foundation, it's estimated as high as 70% of people with dementia are cared for in the home. The caregiver's average age is 51, with about 60% being women.

CHAPTER 13

Paging Doctor Green

The facility's public address system served a variety of purposes. It was used to page people, to make everyone aware of the cookie sale going on to benefit United Way, or to remind everyone of upcoming events. There was also a code used for more serious matters.

"Dr. Red to C Unit," meant C Unit was experiencing a fire. Or, as had always been the case in my experience, a fire drill. I would then be obliged to hustle down there, fire extinguisher in hand.

"Dr. Green, Lower D!" signaled that the staff, almost entirely female, had a problem on their hands and needed help, sooner preferred over later. Patients with aggressive tendencies, suicidal thoughts, or drug and alcohol abuse problems were taken to Lower D, often escorted by officers of the law. The staff on Lower D had extra training specific to the people and situations they dealt with.

Physical confrontation was expected when responding to a Dr. Green page, and employees attended mandatory self-defense classes. The course was given there in the building. A plump matronly female as our instructor did not inspire self-confidence. Besides, I couldn't accomplish a sit-up, so what was I doing on a SWAT team?

"If they grab you by the wrist, you turn this way."

Then, twisting this way and that, she demonstrated what she was talking about. That brought me to the conclusion this wasn't a self-defense class at all. I was learning to square dance.

"If they grab you by the hair, you lean towards them."

We broke off into pairs to practice what we'd just learned, but since I don't have any hair, there was nothing to practice. I'm not aggressive by nature, usually seeking compromise, but with so many of the staff female I felt an obligation to try and help out.

In retrospect, it could be that I didn't take my Dr. Green training as seriously as I should have. However, my experience with Dr. Green episodes taught me that once push came to shove, my defense training flew out the window anyway. I found myself lunging at whatever body part seemed most convenient, content to just hang on. There's incredible difficulty calling to mind your objective was to drain the swamp, when you're up to your ass in alligators.

As is so often the case when experiencing something for the first time, my first Dr. Green call was memorable. For me to reach Lower D, there's a good 100-yard dash involved, and I experienced a level of excitement that, the two added together, kind of took my breath away. Add to that the uncertainty of not knowing what to expect. I'd been warned.

"Expect the unexpected."

But they never said, "*Really unexpected.*"

I busted through the door in my somewhat tentative manner, and was confronted by a young black woman, running right at me, naked as the spot where a pulled tooth once stood. I remembered thinking, "*Now that's odd.*" According to the year 2000 Census, only a half percent of the City's population was African American. I believe the figure rose slightly since then, but still…

There was a voice from somewhere in the back, yelling.

"Grab her!"

"Yes, of course, but *where?*"

The voice was insistent.

"Grab her!"

"I don't think so." My arms hung useless at my sides as she bounced past me, the richness of her voice rang in my ears.

"I'm in Wausau! I'm in Wausau!"

"Me too."

Sadly, however correct, was my only reply. The moment had left me a bit speechless. I'd always championed diversity, and was chagrinned that our chance encounter took place under such regrettable circumstances.

Another early Dr. Green experience involved a young man, in his early twenties perhaps. Very distraught, he was convinced he was dying of cancer at that moment and he needed transportation to the Mayo Clinic, A.S.A.P.

When I arrived on the scene he was standing in the middle of the room surrounded by staff. The charge nurse tried to talk him into medication, but he would have none of it.

"I'll hit the first person that touches me!" he threatened. He was crying, aggressive, and getting more and more out of control.

Once someone got agitated to the point where they broke things, or made threats, there was only one option. Overpower them by sheer numbers and strap them down. People on illegal drugs could demonstrate incredible strength. Remember Dave, the guy who reminisced about Big Johnny? At one Dr. Green call, Dave ended up with a knot on his arm the size of a baseball. On another call, one of our guys had his shirt ripped off, revealing deep, nasty-looking scratches from his neck down to his waistline. I felt bad about that one. In the pile-up, it turned out I had hold of the wrong pair of legs. In effect, I did my best to immobilize the good guy. Personally, I never suffered more than minor bumps and bruises and wounded pride on occasion. I landed on my butt a few times trying to subdue an out-of-control patient a third my age.

We lifted patients, positioned him or her on gurneys, and held them while they were strapped down. Chairs that serve the same purpose are used today. Patients are then rolled into a padded locked room, where they can regain their composure. Not the type of thing I came here to do, I was always left feeling uncomfortable with the entire process.

As we encircled this young man, I felt such empathy. The nurse insisted he make his way to the confinement room, but he wasn't budging and the knot of people around him grew tighter. I felt a sense that if everyone backed off and gave me a minute, I could calm him down. There were too many people, too many orders. Maybe I was naïve. Though I wanted to act on my feelings, I also felt that it wasn't my place. I didn't work on this Unit, never had. With no experience, my feet were locked in cement. The time for talk was over as we all took hold of the guy and strapped him to the gurney. We wheeled him into the room, while he struck out, cried and screamed. I wanted to kick myself for not having the nerve to act on my own. Once he was secured people began leaving, but I stayed behind. I tried to reassure him that everything would be okay. The nurse came in and told me I needed to leave. I didn't doubt her reasoning or qualifications, but in that instant it became clear to me this was a Unit I would never be able to work on.

That said, I responded to a Dr. Green call on a different occasion to find a female staff member sporting a red welt on her cheek, the signs of a black eye already in progress. She was doing her best not to cry, without much success. My attention turned to the offender and out of character, I pushed my way to the front of the line.

During a one week span I answered four or five Dr. Green calls, all for the same individual. He was approximately thirty, with movie star good looks. Trim, fit and muscle-toned, he looked the picture of good health, and like someone who would not take the concept of being strapped down without considerable resistance. Fortunately for all involved, in each instance he eventually reconsidered and made his way on his own to the "quiet room." Though never involved in any life or death struggles with him, he kept me in shape by virtue of having to sprint down to Lower D frequently.

He became disruptive for any number of reasons. One incident I recall had to do with his noon meal, the green beans to be more specific.

I believe he mentioned preferring *"Brussels Sprouts!"*

With that he picked up the entire food tray, and threw it in the general direction of Pittsburg.

During this same time, there was a young woman staying on the Unit. She wore painted-on jeans with holes surrounding both knees. I'd describe her as full-figured. As time went by the young man's condition began to stabilize,

allowing him a certain amount of freedom. I began to notice
the two of them in the hallways together. Soon after, they
were both released. A couple of months later, driving home
through our neighborhood, I saw them peeking through
the window of a house that sported a "For Sale" sign on
the front lawn. I couldn't help but think this whole thing
might be suitable for an episode of "*HOW I MET YOUR
MOTHER.*"

One weekend, we had a Dr. Green alert from the office
of the facility's psychiatrist. I wasn't sure where his office
was, but I knew it was a long way from where *I* was. I also
knew I'd better answer the call. It was a weekend and there
weren't many others around.

After jogging for several minutes I noticed a crowd
gathering down a side hallway and hurried over. I peeked
in the door and began taking mental notes. It was a small
room with a desk, a couple of chairs, and a lamp. Not a lot
of space to roll around in. Sitting on one side of the desk
was the psychiatrist. He looked like he'd eaten something
that didn't sit well. Opposite him was a man I judged to be
in his fifties. Or, was it two men? I wasn't convinced one
man could grow that large.

This individual was very unhappy about something.
My guess was he'd been kicked out of the World Wrestling
Federation for playing too rough. I glanced over my shoulder,
gravely concerned about adequate reinforcements. To my
shock and dismay, it's suddenly apparent I'm the only male
staff that showed up. Another mental note, "*Don't work
anymore weekends.*"

In hostage situations, the experts never act rashly. They
take it slow, feeling time is on their side. That's what began
to unfold as the good doctor put to use all the skills he
could muster.

"*Roger that.*" I was all for, "*Let's talk about this a minute,*" highly doubting the posse gathered behind me would be able to scratch this guy into submission. Eventually, the tension lifted and we were all excused to our various work stations. I arrived on trembling knees, and welcomed the familiar, safe confines of the dementia unit.

There were times people broke chairs apart, wielding the legs around, nails and all. At that point we let the police handle it. They walked in, pulled out the stun gun, and buzzzzzt, just like that, the party was over, and "Thank you all for coming."

According to the American Health Assistance Foundation, Early-Onset Alzheimer's is inherited and rare, affecting less than ten percent of Alzheimer's disease patients. Early-Onset Alzheimer's develops before age sixty-five, in people as young as thirty-five. It is caused by gene mutations on chromosomes one, fourteen, and twenty-one. If even one of these mutated genes is inherited from a parent, the person will almost always develop Early-Onset. All offspring in the same generation have a fifty-fifty chance of developing this type of Alzheimer's if one parent has it. The majority of Alzheimer's cases are late-onset, developing after age sixty-five. There is no known cause, and no inheritance pattern.

CHAPTER

14

The Secret Club

L
inda was a resident of the nursing home at one time, vibrant and outgoing. I remember talking to her in the hallways. Already in her nineties, she bragged about her age, so I was surprised when she was transferred to our unit. Experts say that the tangles and plaques that attack the brain and cause dementia may be present for ten, possibly up to twenty years before outward signs of a problem become apparent. Her longevity may have played a role in tipping the odds against her.

Her family brought in videotapes of Linda leading exercise classes at the retirement home where she once lived. It was fun, remarkable really, seeing her so lively, kicking her feet and shouting instructions. When she came to us, she was still able to talk and still had that twinkle in her eye. Twinkle indeed. It was apparent early on that I had caught Linda's eye. Even with the family there to visit, those eyes followed me wherever I went. She made no attempt to hide her interest.

I had purchased a pair of sunglasses at the Dollar Store, glasses made to humor, ten times the size of a normal pair. Another pair featured the big nose, and bushy mustache. A few residents were beyond noticing, but most would get a chuckle. Not Linda. When I'd walk up to her, a puzzled look would come over her face for a few seconds, but eventually she'd recognize me, despite the get-up.

"You look nice." she'd say. True to her man.

We had a small, soft apparatus the shape and color of a carrot. Many residents balled their hands into fists, exacerbating arthritic conditions. I'd pry fingers open and place the carrot in someone's hands, it helped offset the tension. I had taken Linda aside, rubbing skin cream on her hands and cupping the carrot in her palm. Her eyes locked on me as I tried to help her. The tone of her voice was half wistful, half desperate as she attempted to express her feelings.

"We could put on little black hats and pretend we're typewriters. Oh, I'd like to type with you."

Most Fridays Linda's granddaughter drove all the way from Madison to visit. Linda's daughter, who lived in town, visited several times a week. She came every Wednesday specifically to play the piano for everyone. Devout Catholics, each family member marked the sign of the cross on Linda's forehead before ending a visit. One of their requests was that Linda attend church as often as possible. Her mental health was deteriorating rapidly, possibly because of her advanced age, a mind and body that could no longer fight back. Still, she had been healthy. As she lost more and more control, her strong heart beat on. It reached the point where her vocabulary consisted of just two words, "oh" and "no". She spoke the words in a drawn out manner, each word higher pitched at the start.

"OH-h-h. NO-o-o."

That was Linda's two word response to everything. I never got the impression she spoke out of distress or fear. It was just what she said.

Linda sat beside me in church. I brought a rosary for her to hold. I always enjoyed bringing residents there, regardless of their denomination. Some sat oblivious, while others slept through a whole service. But every now and then, someone's eyes would widen, the wheels in their memory bank trying desperately to turn. It was the lyrics of a favorite hymn, or reciting The Lord's Prayer. Suddenly they'd sit up straighter. Their lips moved, tried to get in sync. Recognition! In a war I knew would one day be lost, it was a victory to savor.

The priest bowed his head then, instructing his faithful to ask forgiveness while calling to mind their sins. The beautiful lady beside me responded the only way she was then capable.

"Oh-h-h. No-o-o."

Linda's daughter died unexpectedly at her home. At the funeral I talked to her granddaughter.

"When the call came in, I assumed it was about grandma. But they said, 'No, we're calling about your mom.'"

I went to a lot of funerals. If they were held in town and I wasn't working, I tried to be there. I didn't usually stay long, but long enough to pay my respects and view the photos. They were like a roadmap of someone's life. When you took care of someone with dementia, someone who was a stranger to you, it could be hard to figure out who they were, and what they must have been like. If they are a person who was hard to deal with, any assumptions were usually negative. And that was not fair. It was like assuming someone with a broken leg was never a fast runner. I went and viewed the photos and gathered as much information as I could about this person I knew. Then I filed it all away for safe keeping. Why, or for how long, I wouldn't know. I guess until it was my turn.

Linda's heart continued to beat, allowing her Alzheimer's to progress to the point where her body began to retract, pulling itself inward. Her hands were balled into fists, tucked under her chin. A few months after her daughter, Linda passed away. She was 100 years old.

༄ ༺

Marvin's wife and daughter visited often and it was obvious they both adored him. You'd think their apparent affection, well earned I'm sure, would register with even a dummy like me.

Not judging a dementia patient by how they acted were easy words to recite, but harder to live by. Marvin was someone I was never able to get close to. Most of what he said didn't make sense, but that's an easy obstacle to overcome once you're used to it. He was perfectly mobile yet refused to take part in any activities, always preferring to keep to himself. He had no real problematic behaviors, but the look on his face always gave me the impression he was up to something. I would converse with Marvin now and then. He was always standoffish, I never felt like I was gaining a sense of trust. That facial expression always left me uneasy.

Then one day it happened. It was mid-afternoon. Snack time. I had a group gathered as I passed out treats. One of the individuals in the group was a man named Fred.

Fred could no longer walk or talk and was seated in his wheelchair. Often when someone passed close to Fred, he would produce a sort of guttural growl. I suppose to someone not familiar it might have sounded threatening, though Fred would be smiling at you seconds later. His growl was simply a "Hi, how are you," Fred style.

Marvin was walking past Fred and was greeted by Fred's standard growl. He jumped back, glared at Fred, and began circling our group. The suspicious look on his face had me keeping a close eye. He'd circled two or three times, when, now directly behind Fred, he bolted forward, grabbed the handles of Fred's wheelchair, and running as fast as he could, escorted Fred in the direction of the nearest wall. Fortunately, I was able to step in front of this two-man parade and bring a halt to it before anyone got hurt. I didn't dislike Marvin, but that one episode reinforced my suspicions—he probably couldn't be trusted.

I attended Marvin's funeral mostly out of respect for the family. I'm glad I went. I saw pictures of Marvin as a younger man, handsome and smiling, that made me swallow. But it was a newspaper clipping about him that really got to me:

'Copters Enter Korean War With Daring Mission

Press reports from overseas credit a Marine helicopter squadron, HMR-161, with accomplishing a first in aviation history in combat this week. They flew in supplies and ammunition to Leathernecks on a ridge on treacherous Korean terrain and evacuated the wounded on the return trip.

HMR-161, formerly stationed at MCAF Santa Ana, is the only Marine helicopter squadron overseas at present.

From dispatches received, they accomplished in one hour with their 10-man "eggbeaters" what 1000 men working a 10-hour day could do. Reports indicate that the higher echelon was impressed with the display and feel it may revolutionize infantry warfare.

Can you imagine? I'd drawn my own conclusions about a man, someone I didn't really know, a person suffering from Alzheimer's, *by the look on his face!* Sometimes, like when I'm about to lose my patience, a tap on the shoulder reminds me of my shortcomings. Then there are times, like at Marvin's funeral, when they march right up and deliver a well deserved slap, right in the face.

❧ ❧

Of everyone I'd met, Gertie owned the cutest smile. It was the dimples that did it.

"What time is it?"

Gertie always asked me what time it was.

"It's 9:00 a.m., Gertie."

She'd always give me a look of disbelief until I assured her it was indeed 9:00 a.m. and then came that little smile that said, "*You're kidding me, right?*" She was so darned cute, I wanted to wrap my arms around her and squeeze all the bad stuff away. Once she was satisfied I was telling her the truth, the conversation moved on for a minute or two, until she would ask again.

"What time is it?"

I never got tired of those dimples.

Gertie was a farmer's wife from the Antigo area. I called her a "potato chip." Antigo is potato farming country, and every time I referred to her this way I got to see those dimples. The Air Force used to have a radar base over that way. While in the Service, when asked where I preferred to be stationed next, my answer was always Antigo. The closest the Air Force came to obliging me was Omaha.

Gertie spent a lot of time in front of our television. She was having a rough time one afternoon, and I surfed the channels for something she might like. I found the show *Animal Planet* just as a mother monkey fed and groomed her baby.

"Look Gertie! See the mother monkey? Isn't that cute?"

I knew she was struggling at the time, but her outraged reply still surprised me.

"I paid good money for that monkey!"

∽ ∾

I arrived at work five to ten minutes early each day and sat in the kitchen trying to get into the right frame of mind. Once I stepped on the Unit I entered a different dimension, and I had to be ready for it. I wanted to be chipper and upbeat. It couldn't matter that the Packers lost or my truck had a flat, the residents deserved more than a push to Bingo.

Unless something else was going on that warranted my attention, I usually started by gathering a group of individuals with appropriate religious backgrounds, and we said the Lord's Prayer. On a personal level I prayed that everyone stayed safe that day, and that I was granted wisdom and patience.

After that, I read the morning paper to everyone, careful to avoid any news items that were shocking or depressing. I passed the paper around for people to read on their own, the ads mostly, but few took advantage. Those who did picked out words here and there, but struggled to ascertain the message given in an entire sentence.

Across the table, Arletta had the newspaper turned to the sports page, which featured pictures of a local bowling tournament. She told everyone about her old job in Milwaukee. That after being promoted to Supervisor, she caught employees stealing. She licked her lips as she always did before she spoke.

"So now they're going to rot in jail forever!" The job, she told us, was at a bowling alley. It won't be long before she'll be repeating the story and Nettie will snap at her,

"You just said that." Nettie recognized and was frustrated by the repetitions of others, though she never realized she, too, was afflicted.

Several residents had therapy appointments. They needed to be taken and picked up at various times. Someone called in sick so we would be a staff member short for awhile. Later there would be a mandatory staff meeting. I hated meetings. Given the choice of a guy in his underwear trying to tip the couch over, or attending a meeting, I'd take the furniture gig every time.

In a few minutes breakfast trays would arrive. We needed to get everyone seated at a table, making sure those seated together got along with each other reasonably well. Once the trays were passed out, and I poured, buttered, cut up, and made everything as ready as possible, I scanned the room, looking for those who were going to need help. Someone who did fine on their own yesterday may not have a clue today.

During this time any number of issues could come up that needed attention. A resident might have something in her mouth that really shouldn't be in there. Arguments, hoarding, wandering, falls or near falls, it wasn't the type of job where you stared at the clock as time dragged by. On any given day, a resident still capable of walking might suddenly appear unsteady. The nurse would warn us to watch that person, ready to assist whenever we noticed them get up. Beside me someone might start to cry. So-and-so was now on thickened fluids. A family was coming to pick up Mom at noon. We would need to have her looking her best and ready to go. *Don't let these two individuals sit near one another...*

And so it went. Another day began. We tried to provide normalcy to a place that was anything but.

I have a couple friends, brothers, whose mother lived there. Nora was a little higher functioning. On a good day she would tell me she knew things were slipping away. She couldn't quite figure it out, but she remembered her life as it used to be, and she missed it. Depression would set in, her illness took charge, and she might start to cry, or become angry. Getting her turned around was not hard.

"Didn't you used to teach Sunday school?"

That was all I had to say. The stories started, and within ten minutes she was singing to me. I worried about when I was no longer there. *Will anyone think to ask Nora about Sunday school?* Perhaps it wouldn't matter. Alzheimer's would eventually take that away from her too. It took until there was nothing left to give. Even at death, it robbed a person. *Shouldn't a person have the right to think? To recognize loved ones? To compose? Summon courage? Shouldn't a person have the right to pray?* I hate this disease.

When I stepped out of the kitchen, I had my game face on as I reminded myself not to lose patience or take things personally. I'd try my best. I knew the challenges I faced today were the same challenges I'd face tomorrow. All I could do was take a deep breath, and reload. Moms and Dads, husbands and wives, had been entrusted to us. This wasn't just a job, it was an honor that insisted on responsibility. I had to remind myself of that sometimes.

For the past week the History Channel featured a series
called *America: The Story of Us.* Featured were events and
people who had shaped our nation. The patients who lived
here were "*us*," too. They came from every walk of life,
every circumstance. People of Negro and Spanish heritage
had slightly higher rates, but other than age, there seemed
to be no correlation. We should all be aware Alzheimer's
may be in our future, or that of a loved one.

Many people fret over a bill they forgot to pay, or
misplaced car keys. They make nervous, half-hearted jokes
about early signs of Alzheimer's. We've all done it. Be more
worried if you find yourself lost in a place that should be
familiar. Are you putting everyday items where they don't
belong? If you have concerns, the best thing to do is get
tested, the sooner the better. You can buy yourself time to
talk with family, plan arrangements, and get your personal
things in the order you want them.

My boss wanted me to start each day with a plan,
a schedule of activities all listed on the black board.
Organization was a skill I'd yet to master, but I tried:
*Devotions at eight o'clock. Exercise after breakfast at nine-thirty.
Grade school kids coming to sing at ten.* Structure was good. I
saw the wisdom there. Then, at 7:59, we'd have a tablecloth
tug of war, and everyone had juice in their lap. At 9:32,
someone's hand touched someone else's shoulder, and I'd
be called in to referee. The kids were into their first song
when one of the guys decided it would be a good time to
take his pants off. Sometimes, when the boss wasn't around,
I slacked off on the planning stuff.

Every week or two the facility brought in musical groups
to entertain the residents. The performances took place
on the nursing home end of the building, so we'd wheel
our people down. The musical group would usually be

a guy, or in some instances, a guy and his wife. The wife wasn't there to help entertain. She lent a hand with the equipment. Once that was accomplished it was her job to sit off to the side and smile proudly. During my time there, the acts were not varied one iota. I knew every song, by every performer, by heart. I'm not afraid to brag here because it was something of an accomplishment when you consider most songs weren't in English. I couldn't speak German or Polish, but I could sing them. The artist almost always wore a funny little hat with a feather sticking out of it. From time to time a little Swiss yodeling was mixed in, which indicated to me that he also sold cough drops. Happy residents laughed, tapped and even yelled.

"Play The Fat Lady Polka!"

I was frozen in a corner praying, *"No, please, not again."*

I didn't mind sitting through these little programs, but it was extremely frustrating to lie down at night, the words to a polka stuck in my head. When finally asleep, I was visited by a very large woman with rosy cheeks. She wore galoshes, cooked giant kielbasas, and prayed to Saint Ladislaus.

∽ ∾

We did not have a Secret Club, so I decided it might be a good idea to start one. Comfortable with smaller groups, I capped the membership at three. And to be fair, I chose members through a lottery drawing I held at my house one night. Gertie, Susan, and Glenda were my chosen victims. I told each a Secret Club had been formed, of which they were now members. With magic marker I applied our "secret sign" to the palms of their hands. Two minutes later no one would remember how it got there. Memory deficiency was key with candidate selection for an organization where secrecy was imperative.

I knew we needed officers. After a lot of thought, I appointed Susan as Recording Secretary; Glenda, Treasurer; with Gertie in charge of Recruitment. I asked if there were any questions. Gertie had one.

"What time is it?"

It was important for Glenda, as Treasurer, to be aware I planned to incorporate a fifty cent fine for anyone found sleeping during a meeting, but I couldn't seem to wake her.

Susan laughed, humored by the whole thing, which was exactly what I had hoped for. She did point out that due to her blindness, her selection as Recording Secretary might need to be revisited. I was forced to tell her to deal with it.

"I'm not changing everything around at this late date."

We had our meetings every afternoon around 2:00 o'clock, and it's hard for me to recall ever having more fun. Laughter was always the order of business, while knowing exactly what it was you were laughing about not being a requirement. Of course, a lot of what went on I'm not at liberty to discuss. It was, after all, a secret club.

I developed a close relationship with Susan. Upon her arrival she suffered from depression, speaking a lot of, "just wanting to die." She refused medication. As she and I grew closer, the nurses took notice. Before long, I was asked if I might be able to get Susan to take her pills. I wasn't allowed to actually dispense anything, but there were no rules against requesting that someone please open their mouth. My success rate with this endeavor was one hundred percent, due solely to the fact that I had the time necessary to gain her trust, and become a friend. I was given a lot of credit where none was due. Once on her medication, the depression ended.

Susan's daughter often sent her mom delicate, handmade greeting cards. I read the cards to Susan, letting her run her fingers over the gentle patterns. We saved all the cards she received, storing them in her bedroom dresser. If she had a bad day, I'd fetch the cards, along with her family album. This always worked wonders. Thinking about it now, I wonder if her daughter was ever made aware of the impact her card creations had on her mom's well being.

As she began to trust me more, Susan, like many other residents, shared her memories with me. She grew up in a small northern Michigan town and moved to Chicago at age eighteen. She found employment, then found love and raised a family. Eventually the family moved back to Wisconsin and opened a tavern.

As time went on, Susan's story changed. Details that once seemed important were left out. Names became puzzles, difficult blurs, mispronounced or conveniently avoided. With Susan and countless others, I had a front row seat at the disintegration of a life story. I tried artfully to remind of important people and events. This proved productive for a while, but the flood waters were building. I knew of no recourse but to sit with them and listen, my thumb against the dyke.

Glenda was not physically imposing, but she was as feisty as they come. Most of the time there were no problems, the exception, her personal cares. Getting dressed, changed, and bathed. These were the times that staff earned their stripes. All CNAs were battle tested. If not, they certainly would be the first time they went in to get Glenda up for the day. With a war going on in the tub room I heard my name yelled, a co-worker needed my help. Glenda liked me, so I was not too concerned there would be a problem. Wrong!

I came out of the tub room looking like I'd just been for a swim, my employee badge broken in half.

I don't recall how it got started, but I began referring to Glenda as a "good looking woman." It became a daily greeting, something I automatically said to her.

"Yur' a good looking woman Glenda."

She would answer me in her squeaky, high- pitched voice.

"Really?"

"Yep."

"No."

"Oh yes, you are."

Her voice would reach new heights.

"Really?"

At her funeral, I learned that Glenda had loved to drink beer, and go fishing. I knew there was something I liked about that woman! This was the kind of personal information that helped so much when someone was in your care. There had always been attempts to gather bits and pieces. A program exists now that does a thorough job of obtaining everything having to do with a person's background, likes and dislikes, work and family history, and religious beliefs.

∽ ∾

It was terribly difficult to watch Gertie decline. It took two of us to help her walk. That precious little face wore a constantly troubled look. In her recliner she fidgeted and fumbled, and tried to slide out entirely, her pant legs rolled up above her knees. She no longer communicated, could not even ask what time it was. Seeing someone you enjoyed in such distress, powerless to do anything about it, was the mother of all dilemmas. She'd freeze in front of me, while I struck matches to the wind. Her stay with us was short. Within a year of her arrival Gertie was gone. At heaven's gate, I hope she smiled.

All of my Secret Club members were gone, their life memberships expired. I'd made feeble attempts to start new secret clubs, but it never worked out. My mind told me it was a good thing to do, but my heart refused to try.

The blessing of this place was that it created so many memories. The curse, no one was a memory until they were no longer with us.

A new lady arrived one day in a wheelchair pushed by her husband. I recognized instantly how protective he was towards her. And, how devastated he felt. I knew how hard it was to bring a loved one here, aware you'd go home alone. At noon I assisted Liz with eating, while her husband held her hand. I sensed she was a woman any husband would be proud to call his own. She spoke, very softly, but only when spoken to. Her eyes were closed, while his eyes spoke volumes. I was looking at someone heartbroken and afraid. From time to time, he scanned the room, taking in the other residents. *Lord, he'd be leaving the love of his life here. What could I say to help him through this? What must he be thinking?* In the background the radio was tuned to an Oldie's channel, Roy Rogers serenaded.

"*HAPPY TRAILS TO YOU!*" I hoped he didn't hear it. The fact that his wife was coming here to live meant we had an open bed, someone else had passed. Any grieving would have to be done at home, off the clock. Right then I had things to do. The place was an emotional roller coaster.

"What can you tell me about your wife?"

He sat up straighter then, I had his attention. With a trembling voice he said,

"Well, she likes classical music….."

He spent the rest of the day sitting with his wife. He was very polite and grateful for any attention given to her by the staff. When supper hour neared, still unable to leave, he ordered a meal for himself. Finally it was bed time. He stood, kissed his wife on the cheek and promised to be back in the morning. Slowly, hesitantly, he made his way toward the door. A condemned man seldom hurries. Like a wavering tree in a barren field, I imagined he faced the strongest wind he'd ever known. This is not how the "Golden Years" were supposed to be. I have never seen another human being looking so completely, utterly alone. At the door he turned for a look back and a final wave. His wife's eyes were closed.

Information supplied by the Centers for Disease Control and Prevention points out the disease has now surpassed diabetes, becoming our nation's sixth leading killer.

CHAPTER 15

Toot Toot

I was working on Side Two of C Unit the day George showed up. Though he was assigned to Side One, I had a chance to meet him briefly during the noon meal. I gauged his dementia to be relatively mild compared to the people he'd come to live with. Confined to a wheelchair, a host of physical problems combined with his confusion, landed him here. His kids were grown and moved away, leaving his wife the sole caregiver. It had become more than she could handle.

The following afternoon, a co-worker from Side One and I took some residents to Bingo on the second floor. There's a large dining room up there, one of the biggest rooms in the building, so it was the place most often used to accommodate large group activities. Getting up there was a bit of a journey. There were two long hallways to travel, an elevator ride, followed by a third hallway, before we reached our destination. Because of the distance involved, even residents who could walk were taken in wheelchairs.

We always took as many people as possible to these events, but the number varied. Some had fallen asleep. When asked, there would be a few who indicated they weren't interested. Others, having a bad day, forced a judgment call as to whether it was practical to include them. I had five or six of my residents up there, and my counterpart from Side One had about the same. George was one of them. My partner and I were both a little worn out and grateful for a chance to sit down. No sooner had we settled in, when George announced that he needed to use the men's room. My co-worker threw me one of those you've-got-to-be-kidding looks. Technically, he wasn't my resident that day, but I thought, what the heck, the guy's gotta go, and I'm young. *What could possibly go wrong?*

There was a bathroom right across the hall, but George was new to me. He was well over two hundred pounds, and I knew nothing of his physical abilities or limitations. *Did his care plan state one person would be sufficient to assist him with this task, or did it dictate two would be necessary?* My only course of action was to take him back to C Unit. Back we went, down the hallway, onto the elevator, and that's where things got interesting.

No sooner did the elevator door close when George immediately began fumbling with his zipper. In the blink of an eye he'd gotten his Johnson whipped out and began doing what came naturally!

"George! STOP!"

"I'm not done yet!"

My hands were tied. "Honest to GOD!"

I must have been asleep in class when they explained what to do when your resident is taking a piss on the elevator. I envisioned our coming to a stop, the door opening to three little old ladies, mouths agape, palms pressed to their hearts. Maybe they'd decide to sue me for not preventing this horror they'd been forced to witness. The State would get involved, and levy a stiff fine against the nursing home, forcing the facility to close its doors. Families in the Tri-County area we served would be left without a much needed resource. With my employment gone, I'd fall behind on mortgage payments, my marriage collapsing under the strain. Maggie would remarry a yoga instructor from Chippewa Falls—and all because some guy I just met had to take a leak! Over the public address system a message seldom heard.

"Housekeeping to the elevator. STAT!"

Funny, ain't it? How things could happen I mean.

Over time I got to know George a lot better, that he had a very friendly, gentle disposition. Another retired farmer, a life's work he confessed had always been a struggle.

"Damned rocky ground. No good," he'd say, shaking his head.

When he told me where his homestead had been, I mentioned that I owned a little land out in that general direction. As his confusion progressed, he took my bit of information and convinced himself that we had farmed near one another. He started calling me Chucky.

"Chucky boy, how's yer hay comin' this year?" he'd want to know.

One day he asked, "Chucky boy, remember that time when you and me was at Lakeview Ballroom?"

Slapping his knee and laughing hard, I was forced to reminisce, without the benefit of ever having actually been there. A veteran, husband, father, and finally, a resident here. Life's steps didn't always lead up.

I learned one more thing about George. He was on fluid
restrictions. Bladder problems.

∽ ∾

With so many people in wheelchairs, it was tough
figuring out how to get everyone any exercise. It helped to
be creative. I'd strung everyone out in a straight line and
explained that they were now a train. I had Roy in front, the
engine. I barely knew what he looked like. He was forever
complaining of being cold, so the majority of the time he
was covered in blankets from head to toe.

"I want a fire." Roy told me one morning.

Assuming he was still cold, I went and got another
blanket.

"I don't want that!" he yelled.

"I want a fire! I'm gonna roast a pig!"

Rosie was on the other end, the caboose. The image
struck her fancy. And that was good, because Rosie was
someone who could make or break whatever you were
trying to do so her willing participation was key.

"The rest of you guys are passenger cars and we've got a
long way to go, so let's start moving like a train, okay?"

I'd pump my arms, chug-a-chug-a, chug-a-chug-a.

"Come on you guys. Pump your arms, chug-a-chug-a."

My caboose grinned and worked away, but the rest of
the train was apparently on strike. I pumped and chugged
and implored, with no results. My little experiment seemed
destined for failure and I was about to give up, when, from
under a pile of blankets…movement! Seconds later there
was a piercing.

"Woo! Woo!"

My engine kicked in! Another pair of arms started chugging, and before we knew it we were rolling! It's such a small, silly thing. But everyone laughed. Everyone had a good time. They even got a little exercise.

Roy could get pretty confused, but I never doubted his recollections about some things. He shared stories of being in World War II and how he was wounded.

"I got shot in the ass in New Guinea!"

Often, his memories brought tears. But not that day. That day we were *'ridin' on the City of New Orleans, and we'd be gone five hundred miles for the day is done.'*

"Woo! Woo!"

A little postscript about Roy and his war recollections: I've just finished reading *The Ghost Mountain Boys* by James Campbell, about the God-awful World War II, South Pacific battle for Papua New Guinea. Gaining control of the island allowed our bombers access to the Japanese homeland. I highly recommend this insightful, thoroughly researched work, which has provided me an entirely new perspective, and a deep sense of gratitude for all who served there. Where would we be today had it not been for men like Roy? I've come to realize that under our pile of blankets was an American hero.

✧ ✧

I'd spent the better part of an hour getting a dozen or so people stationed around our large circular table. Trying to get dementia patients organized took a little effort. You can't just yell, "Hey everybody, c'mere a minute!" Anyway...
"I thought we might do a little singing, so listen up you

guys. I'm going to start singing a song, okay? And when I raise my arms, you guys all sing 'Toot-Toot!' okay?"

It was a good group, everyone smiling and nodding in agreement.

"Okay, here we go." I began to sing.

"She was born in her birthday suit! The doctor slapped her behind! He said you're gonna be special, you sweet little—" I raise my arms and—nothing.

"Come on you guys, you missed your cue! When I raise my arms you all sing 'Toot-Toot!' okay?"

Everyone smiled and nodded in agreement.

"Let's try it again. She was born in her birthday suit! The doctor slapped her behind! He said you're gonna be special, you sweet little—" I raise my arms and—nothing.

Good grief. A half dozen or so more attempts, everyone continued to smile and nod in agreement, and—nothing.

"Listen guys, you can do this. I know you guys can toot, I've heard you!"

Everyone smiled and nodded in agreement. *One last time.*

"She was born in her birthday suit! The doctor slapped her behind! He said you're gonna be special, you sweet little—" I raise my arms and—Emma squeaks.

"Toot-Toot!"

"YES! ALRIGHT! Did you hear that guys? Emma tooted! This time I want you all to join in. When I raise my arms, you all sing 'Toot-Toot!' just like Emma did. Okay?"

Everyone smiled and nodded in agreement.

"Here we go! She was born in her birthday suit! The doctor slapped her behind! He said you're gonna be special, you sweet little—" I raise my arms and—Mildred croaks.

"Toot-Toot!"

"YES!" But I lost Emma. This was going to be harder than I thought.

"Listen you guys, we can do this. I know it. Wait for the part where I raise my arms, then you all sing 'Toot-Toot!' right?"

Everyone smiled and nodded in agreement.

One more last time. "She was born in her birthday suit! The doctor slapped her behind! He said you're gonna be special, you sweet little—" I raise my arms and—Lynette belts out...

"ARMS!" And I lost Emma and Mildred. Maybe I pushed too hard.

Complications of Alzheimer's disease include: Loss of ability to care for oneself, inability to interact, malnutrition and dehydration, failure of body systems, harmful or violent behaviors, falls and broken bones.

CHAPTER 16

The Deer Hunt Gang

Some people you had to learn to like. With Sid, you were pretty much hooked from the get-go. He was a man of many hats. Literally. He stacked them one on top of the other, then put the whole shebang on. I personally saw him with as many as four at a time but heard his record was six. It would be a collage of whatever he discovered was available, from a woman's chapeau to baseball caps, Sid should have been an engineer. It was like viewing new age art work.

If the Unit was a jungle, Sid was our lion. When he started giving orders, we had to listen close, he sounded like someone struggling to swallow an octopus. His wife and son came nearly every morning to feed him breakfast. For them he would pretty much eat everything, but once they were gone he wouldn't touch anything except chocolate ice cream. Much of Sid's day was spent asleep in a recliner. An oxygen machine sat next to his throne. If he started turning purple we hooked him up.

Sid should have been in Congress. I'd never heard anyone talk so much without ever getting anything accomplished. If not Congress, what about a radio talk show host? He'd be the perfect sidekick for Rush (me to the hospital) Limbaugh.

It was hard to pick up the gist of Sid's dissertations. The line of snot dangling precariously from his nose reached a length so impressive, it joined in wedlock with the saliva overflow created by the bubble machine inside his mouth, thus creating world class distraction. Don't try bringing a towel to clean him up; Sid didn't appreciate being interrupted when he was onto something.

While he enjoyed an audience, it was not a necessity. Sid gargled away at imaginary crowds, too. He'd be asleep in his chair for over an hour, then wake suddenly, and begin giving hell to the thin air surrounding him. One afternoon he was at it again and kept it up, making such a ruckus, that I went over to see what the problem was. A little back rubbing and affirmation that I agreed with him on all counts usually calmed him down. His ranting was pretty unintelligible, but once he started to ease off I was able to pick up this much.

"I like women, I really do."

Sid was just a little guy, not a whole lot over five feet tall. His normal weight was around 130, but that could balloon quite a bit. It all depended on what he had in his pockets. When Sid was up and about, he did a lot of shopping. In and out of other residents' rooms, opening closets, shuffling through drawers. It was all done in an orderly manner, Sid was in no rush. If he came across a necklace that caught his fancy, he'd spend a half hour examining, pouring it back and forth, one palm to the other. Eventually, he came to a decision. Sale or no sale. No sale, he tossed it back in the drawer. Sale, he shoved it in his pocket. No money ever exchanged hands.

The Unit was Sid's oyster. In the past, the CNAs forever chased him out of other people's rooms, wrestling away his treasures. But it was bothersome for the staff, and more importantly, upsetting to Sid. Now they allowed him to shop. When they got him ready for bed at night, they'd empty his pockets *and* the hats, there was stuff in there, too. They did their best to put it all back where it belonged. On a good shopping day, Sid hauled in jewelry for sure, dentures, maybe a toothbrush, a bra that would never fit, a picture of someone in a Santa Claus suit, and a chocolate bar that melted three hours prior. One bite missing. And hats.

~∾ ℘~

If you want good venison sausage, you have to come to Wisconsin. If you want great venison sausage, you have to go to a little butcher shop in Mosinee where I used to go. Until it closed. The owner retired. He locked the door and walked away without so much as a 'Here's the recipe!' It took me years to find another place that offered anything nearly as good.

As it turned out, one of the guys on E Unit, Lee, was my retired butcher! I stumbled across this bit of information while talking with his daughter. She told me he never wrote the recipe down, it was always in his head. He was a pleasant, gentle, agreeable man. When he died, a lot of people at the funeral wondered why his final years had to be spent as an Alzheimer's patient. And why he never wrote the damn venison sausage recipe down.

Deer hunting in this part of the country is an honored tradition. Employers field calls from ill employees while teachers instruct half empty classrooms. Some even refer to the season as 'Holy Week.' Maggie thinks I'm a fanatic. Originally from Illinois, I'm not sure she understands. Still, I've been known to get up at one o'clock a.m. on opening day of each season, unable to sleep. Travel time is not the problem. I hunt a half-hour from home. Decades ago I wrote an essay for my own pleasure, and to put the sport into perspective for an outsider. I titled it *The Gift.* It reads as follows:

My first deer season, so long ago, my dad whispered in my ear, "Charlie, its 4:30, time to get up son."

Yesterday escapes on eagles wings, but I still remember. I grudgingly got out of bed that morning, put on the brand new pair of long-johns laid out for me the night before, wondering if anything could be worth getting up for at such an early hour.

The days and weeks previous had been building with anticipation, but with an equal supply of self doubt. I harbored a deep concern any silly mistakes on my part might ruin Dad's deer season. I shouldn't have worried. The nine days of that November season, and the Novembers to follow, would bond us like no other time.

Stumbling into the kitchen that morning I was entering a world new to me. Left behind were cartoons, footballs and reading assignments. I never missed them. I was introduced to bacon tasting better than it ever had before. To the odor of gun oil and old wool. To the feel of sharp knives. I met big men with beards who would soon become my heroes. To biting cold, snow storms, leg cramps, swamps and stumps, rocks, hills, gullies, thorns, rabbits, eagles, hawks, porcupines, raccoons, foxes, grouse, and one year when the lake had yet to freeze over, thousands of ducks, so many they blackened the sky. Along with all these, the magnificent whitetail deer.

Oh the memories. Seeing Dad in those goofy pants he always wore. They billowed at the sides, like Sgt. Preston of the Yukon used to wear, then laced with strips of leather at the calf, skin tight. Seeing him in those things I'd try desperately not to laugh, scared to death he'd be angry, or even worse, hurt. Learning to field dress my first deer.

"You want me to cut off his what?!"

I was supposed to be in school the day I got my first buck, a circumstance that agitated Mother to no end. Though Dad was a thoughtful, loving husband, when the subject was deer hunting, she knew to tread lightly.

Deer season provided a different picture of Dad. His mood, habits and daily routine changed. He was excited! A guy who never talked on the phone was now dialing long distance! Hunting stories were being told. They didn't make a lot of sense to me at the time, but I filed them away for safe keeping. Today I can see them in my mind's eye as if I had actually been there when they took place. I could sense the anticipation building in my dad, spilling over until it was rubbing off on me, a little boy who was just beginning to learn what this time was all about.

Seeing him though, kneeling over a fallen buck, his nose running, holding his bad hand that pained him so in the cold, there was a glint in his eye and flush on his cheek reserved for only this time in November.

Opening day included a trip to the tavern at day's end. More Pepsi's and Snicker's bars coming my way than I could ever have imagined. Seeing my dad, the stoic rock who resided in our living room, laughing at the bar. The newspaper I was accustomed to seeing him hold replaced by a shot of brandy. To a twelve- year- old this may not have been heaven, but I felt a strong sense we were getting close. I wanted to throw my arms around Dad and tell him I loved him. That, of course, was something men, even men in the making, didn't do.

Eventually the tavern phone would ring, Aunt Leona alerted us.

"Supper is on the table!"

But my aunt had been through this before. In truth, she had hardly begun preparations, well aware it would take some time to separate this bunch from their surroundings. Like a farmer plans fall harvest, she was merely planting the seed.

Once the meal had been enjoyed the men would begin planning the next day's hunt, something they had already gone over several hundred times while still at the tavern. Personally, I would begin a losing battle to keep my eyes open. Soon, visions of a whitetail giant would be dancing in my head. As I nodded off to sleep, I was beginning to understand why these nine days in November were so special.

A lot of deer seasons have come and gone since then. Dad's gone, too. There's no one to wake me now when it's time to get up. No one has to. Not all of Dad is gone though. His 1892 lever action Marlin 32 Special, the only rifle the man ever owned, waits patiently for its next season in a place of honor, over the fireplace. That gun means the world to me. His ancient Western pocket knife rests in my dresser drawer, sharp as the day it was born. Dad's old, red wool hunting jacket, all battered and torn, hangs with my hunting clothes, and there it will stay. My most treasured possessions are the memories.

These are the things my father left me: A rifle, a knife, some warm clothes and warmer memories. But these are things any son might expect. I received something else from him though. A gift. You can't see it, or taste it, or hold it in your hand, but it's as real as a Father's love. It is an indescribable love and respect for hunting, for nature and the out-of-doors, and for the magnificent whitetail deer.

I wanted to, had to, write this little story for a couple of reasons. First, because I'm not sure I ever took the time to say, "Thank you, Dad."

Second, because this season will be special for me. Oh, I imagine on opening morning I'll be getting up at the usual time. I'll get the

coffee going and wash up a bit. But then! Then I'll tip-toe to the
upstairs bedroom, crack open the door and whisper,
    "Kelly, it's 4:30, time to get up son."

෧ ౿

I considered the notion of having a deer hunt right there on the Unit. With our resident population predominately female, I was concerned I might not be paying enough attention to the guys. There were a number of reasons for the gender disparity. For one, Alzheimer's is age driven and women live longer.

I asked Sid's wife if her husband had been a deer hunter. With ten guys to choose from I was certain there'd be some hunters in the bunch. I wouldn't include someone with no past interest, so I made inquiries. She answered yes, Sid had been a deer hunter, but she had put an end to it. Curious, I asked why. The look on her face reminded me of the hell-hath-no-fury expression. She explained about the morning Sid and his brothers were out the door for a day of deer hunting at Nine Mile. Nine Mile is a large tract of woodland not far from town. Crisscrossed with biking and ski trails, it's a favorite destination for hunters as well.

Apparently, after leaving the house, the brothers came up with a new plan. Instead of Nine Mile, they decided to head "Up North."

Oh boy, I pictured this already. The day had passed with no word. As darkness fell, she felt a little worried. They were usually home by now. Hours passed, and a little worry turned to real concern. When she could wait no-longer she phoned the authorities, and it was right about then Sid and his brothers-in-arms came stumbling in.

"We were on our way home from Up North," Sid explained with a nervous grin, "everyone battling a great thirst when, mother of all blessings, we located a tavern and—"

And that was the last time Sid went deer hunting. Proof: If momma ain't happy, ain't nobody happy.

౿ఎ ౿ఎ

I spend many days in the deer woods. Not only with a rifle but with a bow as well. Being in the woods grounds me and provides time to reflect. I know how valuable time spent among the trees can be to someone with the forest in their blood. Sometimes while hunting my mind took me back to the nursing home and the people I helped take care of. I thought of the family albums, often filled with hunting and fishing photos. Scenes these people will never realize again. Thinking about them, I sometimes felt depressed. But, there's a cure out there, a lot of smart people, working hard. I've had to remind myself of that. A man will never see the horizon if he's forever staring at his feet. Yet donations for Alzheimer's research lags far behind totals given towards cures for other major diseases.

౿ఎ ౿ఎ

I'd rounded up a respectable number of guys for our deer hunt, and showed up at work with every piece of hunting equipment I owned, minus the guns. Compasses, binoculars, a couple of rifle scopes, buck grunts, doe bleats, antlers for rattling, and a lifetime worth of blaze orange hats. I also brought a section of rope, and a life-sized deer decoy.

Before long we were on the lookout for a big one. We rattled the horns, blew the buck grunts, wheezed the doe bleats, and made tasteless remarks whenever one of the girls walked by, because that's what you do when you're deer hunting. Finally I knocked the decoy over and with all the excitement I could muster I hollered.

"Eddie, you got him! Way to go Eddie!"

Eddie is a character. His wife told me about the day she arrived for a visit and asked her husband, "Do you know my name?" Eddie asked her, "Don't *you* know it?"

Eddie looked a little puzzled about his sudden hunting success, but after a couple of hand shakes and slaps on the back he was buying in. Dragging a deer out of the woods is hard work, but Eddie's sons had told me their dad had hunted for years, that he was a good hunter, tireless and willing. Which is probably why, when I asked Eddie if he would help me drag the deer out, he let out a deep exhale before answering with a determined tone, "Well, lets get it over with."

Eddie's ability to comprehend had been ravaged. His days were spent lost in a world known only to him, yet for an hour or two we'd found a way to bring him closer. Yogi Berra knew what he was talking about when he said, "It ain't over til it's over."

We dragged Eddie's prize around the Unit for all to see, eventually hanging it up so pictures could be taken. It was a special moment, but not my favorite part of the day. My favorite part had come earlier, while passing out the blaze orange hats.

Ned was young when he came to us, in his early sixties. He was tall, handsome, and built like a linebacker, still able to walk and talk back then. He'd been a fireman, with a look and demeanor that gave me visions of him geared up, emerging from smoke and flame with a baby under each arm. He was in a body length wheelchair now, his face expressionless. If asked a question, there was seldom a response. On his best day you might get a "Yep."

Alzheimer's played with some, taking its time. With others it was in a hurry. Once symptoms appeared, the average life expectancy for Alzheimer's patients is eight years. With Ned it was in a rush, a little more of him disappeared each day. But I'd been told that he had loved to deer hunt! I waved a blaze orange hat in front of his face, yelling about deer hunting. I asked excitedly if he was coming along. Ned's eyes opened wide, his face stretched in anticipation. A man who no longer talked managed to say,

"Yeah, let me go get my..." before his voice trailed off and his face went blank. Not much of a thing some might say. But I say, for a few seconds Ned had a special time in his life back. That was my favorite part.

That night I watched as a couple of the girls emptied Sid's pockets and hats, ready to tuck him in. He protested a little, dragging his feet like he sometimes did, but I wasn't worried. He'd had a long day of hunting, so I was confident. The lion would sleep tonight.

A person with Alzheimer's disease will live an average of eight years and as many as twenty years or more from the onset of symptoms.

Final Thoughts

I haven't always been conventional around the nursing home, there have been times my antics drew some questionable looks. A line from an old Waylon Jennings song seemed to suit me: *'I've always been crazy but it's kept me from going insane.'* Around here, laughter and despair are forever butting heads. In order to survive, I had to let the good times win.

Large group activities could be a lot of fun, but my female co-workers were better at organizing those types of events. Being alone with a patient where I could try to calm and communicate was what I found most rewarding. When I first started working on the dementia unit I arrived with good intentions but few skills. I remember being uncomfortable at the thought of holding another man's hand. That sounds ludicrous but it was a small hurdle, one of many, I needed to overcome. I've learned about the healing power of the human touch and that my inhibitions made me less of a person.

The patio behind North Central Health Care offers a panoramic view of Lake Wausau. A favorite place to visit, I've been there too many times, with too many people. Out on the lake boats pass by, their wakes break against the shore, pounding, slapping, before diminishing, until you're left with only the memory. Not unlike a life.

If it's been a good day, I walk home past flower gardens, dogs racing after Frisbees, kids on bikes, the odor of charcoal burning. But on days where another bed rests, empty and waiting, it's a journey through a grey tunnel. Emotional closeness, caring *about* people, not just for them, is that double-edged sword that carries me through the stresses this place can offer up. And falling on your own blade is common, the reason so many leave this field. Henry David Thoreau was right, "The heart is forever inexperienced." Each time you lose someone, the more you've cared, the more you're left bloodied. Some residents pass away before you get the chance to know them, or get acquainted with the family. It may seem a minor thing, until you recognize it for what it is. Not a singular occurrence. It visits you again, over and over. You can tell yourself it's of little matter, that strangers' tears won't affect you. But your heart learns the truth. I could handle the bizarre situations, the confounding behaviors, even the failures I experienced. I wasn't prepared for the loss I would feel. Away from the nursing home I can go about my life, feeling sorry for myself if I've a mind to, while those living with Alzheimer's stay frozen in time. They have no past to call their own, and no promise of a brighter tomorrow.

A bed never stays empty for long. The greatest risk factor for developing Alzheimer's is advancing age, and we've reached a point in time where baby boomers have arrived. According to Snapshot, 2009-2011 Edition, a brochure that provides statistics concerning life here in Marathon County, in 2008, 13.7% of the County's population was 65 or older. That number is projected to be 23% by 2030. North Central Health Care can accommodate over seventy patients on its dementia units. There are other capable facilities in our area as well, yet the waiting lists continue to grow.

Faith can leave me like a kite to the wind. The memories pile up, like photos in an album, until there's no more room. The little bird that once sang on my shoulder as I turn my album's pages becomes an albatross, telling me, "*You can't do this forever.*"

The screams from someone down the hall go unheard, yet nights are visited by the murmurs of someone who sat next to me that day, just trying to endure. Faith will return I know, when my complaining has stopped, but from my house I can hear the sirens. My mind questions, who this time, my stomach sours, and before I know it, here I go again, dancing with the devil.

My time at North Central is getting short. As I write this, I'm days from retirement. I'm sixty-two, with places that itch. I figure best to get them scratched while I can still reach.

To a lesser degree, but still pertinent in my retirement decision, is the job description I now have. When I was moved to C Unit my former position was eliminated, and I was officially assigned to the activities department. On my former Dining and Transport job I spent most of my time with the residents. Transfer to the activities department seemed a natural fit. But activities have been going through expansion, with specific goals in mind. That being the case, it's somewhat regimented.

The first thing every morning, we list all the activities planned for the residents that day. We always include as many people as possible. There's documentation to fill out.

In the past, I'd been an activity department unto myself, forever adlibbing, goofing around with whatever came to mind. Attempting to plan eight hours of goofing around is something I found difficult. In addition, I'd always been most comfortable in one-on-one situations, or with small groups. I would grab a couple of aprons for instance, and select someone to help me dust the place. With someone in a wheelchair, I'd give them the handle of the vacuum cleaner, and then push them around the Unit, a two-man suction team. It was fun and meaningful, but a far cry from including everyone.

Before my twenty-seven years at UPS, I spent six years working at a paper mill. Before that it was four years with Uncle Sam. In each situation the majority of co-workers were men. At the nursing home it was just the opposite, something I struggled with. My dilemma can be explained in one word. Drama. Drama-drama-drama. Constant! Someone was forever whispering some deep, dark secret in my ear before scurrying off to unload on the next person. My co-workers were good people who loved the residents, better than I was at entertaining large groups, but I could never get them to understand, *I don't give a crap what Susie said to Jackie when she found out Jenny was pregnant and it might be Billy's but maybe not and her car's not even paid for and now she may have to move back home and she'll have to watch her diet and that'll be really hard and Billy said he's not even sure he likes her because she talks so much and now he's letting his hair grow long and it looks really stupid and he can be a real jerk but she thinks he's so cool just because he bought her a cat and O.M.G. what if the baby's allergic and if they get engaged we should throw them a big party and don't tell anybody!* Constant.

We had monthly meetings that were kind of, sort of mandatory. But I didn't attend. I did go once, but left early. I was the only male in the bunch. We were supposed to banter ideas around, but before there was time to even scratch my head, I found myself in a hail storm. Someone should have passed out napkins. These women salivated over the concept of being paid to talk. I was quickly overwhelmed. The closest thing to an idea I had was,

"Who's with the residents while we're all in here bantering?" So I left.

No one has ever directed me to better adapt, but I felt a certain pressure and a sense that I'd lost my edge.

The very last Dr. Green alert I answered gave me some self satisfaction. Earlier in the day there had been a call concerning this individual, but at the time I'd been outside with a resident, leaving me unavailable to help. One of the guys who answered the page told me there'd been quite a tussle. When I arrived on the scene, the individual sat on the edge of his bed, very upset, refusing to budge. The Unit staff quickly surrounded him.

"Don't get too close," they warned.

By now I had enough experience with Dr. Green's that I felt comfortable telling myself, *The hell with it, for once I'm going to try this my way.* I sat down on the bed next to the guy, started talking, and a few minutes later he and I walked hand in hand to the quiet room. If there is such a thing as a good Dr. Green call, in my mind, that was it.

Of the nine students in my CNA class, only two remain. And once I'm gone, one. I don't know what became of them. Some went on to become nurses. On E Unit recently, I did a little head count. Of the twenty-six residents living there when I first arrived, only two remained. That doesn't take into account the many that came after I started, and since passed on. I confess I can't remember them all, at least not all the names. With my eyes closed, struggling to recall, some of the faces appear with perfect clarity, while others drift by like images in a faded mirror. I'm certain if I were to somehow view a list, it would put me in a nostalgic tailspin.

Leaving will be bitter sweet. I listened as a football coach tried to explain his mixed emotions. He was leaving the school he'd been at for many years to pursue a better offer.

"It's like watching your mother-in-law drive over a cliff, in your brand new Cadillac Escalade."

I know I'll go over to the nursing home from time to time, just to say hi and mingle with the residents. As a matter of fact prom night is coming up. I've got a hot date with a lady from Upper D. Not a solitary soul will remember me, but that's okay. I'll put my arms around every single one and say,

"But I remember you."

One of our residents had two daughters. Elsie's dementia was severe, and had been for quite some time. The first daughter came nearly every day, and had done so for nearly a decade. Her visits were not the pop-in variety. She questioned the nurses, wanting assurances Mom's needs were met. They took walks together. She set her mother's hair. This daughter took laundry home, returned it neatly pressed, and arranged on hangers in the order she would like to see everything worn. The second daughter visited perhaps two or three times a year, insisting it was too difficult seeing Mom in her condition. I could appreciate that. I had empathy. But those who stared this disease in the eye, refusing to blink, earned my deepest respect.

Three women showed up one day to visit an old friend. As they were leaving, one of them took me aside. She seemed indignant.

"I don't think we'll come again," she told me. "She doesn't recognize us. I don't think she even knows we're here."

It was as if they had performed an obligation and the matter was now taken care of. The fear of Alzheimer's directs us to distance ourselves, not learn more. Yet, those afflicted have no resource without the convictions of others. I know it wasn't that these women didn't care, they simply lacked the will. We need to summon courage and follow where our hearts lead us. Without courage, all other virtues are useless.

When family or friends visited, especially if they didn't come often, some easily fell into the common sense trap. If the person with Alzheimer's said something outrageous like...

"My mother's coming to pick me up!"

"Your mother's been dead for years!" was a reaction that arose from frustration. Or, "How old is your mother now?"

It must be remembered, don't argue, and don't contradict.

"Tell me about your mother," would be a more appropriate response.

If you've considered a visit to someone, but aren't sure, by all means do it. Bring a snack along, but check with the nurse before handing anything out. Bring family pictures. You never know when a photo or familiar phrase may trigger a positive reaction. Most importantly, bring your memories. And treat someone the way you hope to be treated.

I watched a large group of family members, upset with their mom, who refused to take her medication. The longer it went on, the more out of control things got. What started out as suggestions, turned to directions, then to actual threats. Voices rose.

"Take your pills or we won't visit anymore!"

I tried to calm things down but realized Mom would not be taking any pills, she was far too upset. Too many people spoke at once. Too many orders. We had to appreciate how overwhelming it must be for someone making an effort just to put one foot in front of the other.

If you come to visit, go with the flow. Let any conversation take you where it will, you can still discover the person you once knew and loved. They are still there, hiding behind a wall of confusion. It's best to figure out a way around, not a way to blast through.

Some lived there for years. If they had a family who visited often, I became a part of that life story. The guy who helped care for Mom or Dad, a husband or wife. I found myself invited to an inner circle, often included in private matters. It wasn't something taught in class, but was, without a doubt, part of the job. Then, just as we'd all get comfortable they'd be gone and a new family arrived. The cycle started over. I began by welcoming them to the neighborhood.

"Hi, I'm Chuck. What can you tell me about your Mom?"

Some people would be tentative at first, but most times information gushed out like a dam burst. Fears, angers, frustrations. The overwhelming feeling of helplessness.

"She was a wonderful cook. Mom loved to sew." Mom might be sitting two feet away yet they spoke in past tense. "Dad built his own house." Stories that had become all too familiar. Often tears would start as I was handed the keys to someone else's life. I'd come a long way since that first day with Mabel, and learned a lot about what it meant to be human. Caring and friendship were sacred medicine. With faith, for every loss there was spiritual consolation.

I leave there certain my life has been enriched. I received more than I gave. My time there doled out countless frustrations and painful losses, but when I close my eyes and think of Sally, making beds and singing our songs together, and so many others, my heart smiles. The good from all of this was worth any injury, great or small.

I often heard apologies from the families of those living with Alzheimer's. People tried desperately to excuse the behavior of a loved one whose mind had been set adrift. I hope this book reaches you. I hope to convey a message. *There are people who understand. Your loved one, regardless of his or her dementia, is capable of being loved by someone who up until now was a stranger.*

What started as a retirement job, turned into a love affair. At my little retirement party I talked with Lori Koeppel, the nursing home Director, a woman who rescued the facility from the financial brink. She's the person responsible for numerous improvements to the home's quality of care. Still a young woman, her accomplishments have established a reputation for success.

I asked Lori about her plans for the future, expecting to hear comments about advancement and opportunities. She answered that her dream was to one day purchase a small farm. Then to construct a home, where she could bring maybe fifteen or so of "her guys" to live. She pictured a place where the men could use their hands again, work with the land, and ultimately, regain self-worth. When it came to love affairs, I wasn't the only one.

I'm no theologian, sure as hell no saint, but I know when something feels good. From day one, this job felt good. Someday history teachers will remind students of a time when there were nuclear bombs, oil spills, racism, and dreaded diseases. I don't believe God is waiting for us to finally screw up royally—He's waiting for us to finally get it right.

I'd asked many residents "Are you an angel? Were you sent down from above to test us?"

No one ever admitted to it. The one word Frieda ever uttered to me was, "Philadelphia."

But still, I've got my suspicions. How else can you explain feeling richer the more you give?

A teacher asks his class, "Which is the greater concern, not having knowledge, or not having empathy?"

A student answers, "I don't know, and I don't care."

For those residing in nursing homes and regarding those with dementia in particular, ignorance isn't bliss. It's the easy gate. The opposite of love is indifference. Don't get caught one day being judged on your neutrality.

Earlier, I alluded to a nursing home as a person's last resort. In my mother's case, I knew that to be true. But my pen was too caught up in my own personal drama at the time. People arrive at nursing homes for all sorts of reasons, horrid misfortune, or crippling circumstance. Many have years to live, and despite every effort, they can be lonely.

Mother Teresa said, "Loneliness and being forgotten are the two greatest poverties."

Family, friends, clergy, a caring staff, and volunteers all play a role in adding quality of life for nursing home residents. People who care are building blocks to self-esteem and a life worth living.

We had a lot of kids visit, not just family members, but school groups, from high school choirs to pre-school. As soon as children walked in the door, you'd see a motherly instinct kick in with nearly all of our women. Their efforts could be awkward, but they still attempted what came naturally. One of our guys, Fred, cried whenever kids showed up. Fred couldn't tell us what was wrong, but it happened every time. His tears said what his voice couldn't.

This is a wonderful place to volunteer. If you know how to talk, how to listen, you qualify. The elderly don't seek miracles, or a new lease on life. They need a reason to wake up tomorrow. That's not a lot to ask. An old man will talk about yesterday, an old woman, about today. And with that, life endures. At church one Sunday our Pastor talked about the virtues of service to others. He asked how many in attendance that day had ever done any volunteer work. He began reciting a long list of facilities and organizations.

"Raise your hand if you have ever helped any of the following. Hospitals, nursing homes, The Salvation Army, United Way, Big Brothers Big Sisters…"

All around me, hands were going up, many repeatedly. It's a wonderful feeling, being surrounded by heroes.

I stated earlier the people described in this book are real, and the events herein actually took place. Truth is, indeed, stranger than fiction. But my descriptions were not just an effort to keep readers entertained. It is how I dealt with things, my life raft in an often stormy sea. That is the only bit of evidence I know to submit as to this work's truthfulness.

By the year 2029, all Baby Boomers will be at least age sixty-five. Projection: Six hundred and fifteen thousand new cases a year.

CHAPTER 18

The Answer

A nurse told me it was a medical condition that caused Elsie's lower lip to hang down so much. Her constant drooling was the first thing you noticed. Nearly always on the move, Elsie was in and out of other residents' rooms, always searching, never finding. Six out of ten people affected by Alzheimer's will wander. If you were seated somewhere, it was only a matter of time before you felt Elsie standing over you, a thin line of drool dangling precariously over your head. We tucked a washcloth in her shirt, just below her chin. When I first came here, it was this condition that kept me literally at arm's length for some time. A long gone prejudice of mine.

She was tall and thin, her face gaunt. She made sounds and gestures, but her ability to speak had left her. I had known her for five years, and she never said a word. Elsie had her likes and dislikes. Once, I made the mistake of saying good morning to her while one of the girls was putting curlers in her hair. I ended up with a glass of orange juice in my face. Elsie didn't appreciate getting her hair fixed.

I don't know what I expected the first time I gave her a hug, but as I put my arms around her and kept them there, she gave a soft whimper, as if it was something she had sorely needed. My attachment to her was instantaneous, and set in stone.

Elsie didn't take part in any activities except music. Smiling and laughing, her feet tapped and her arms danced to the rhythm. The only other tool that helped her get through the day was her doll. If you got her seated and handed her that doll, she might find respite from her endless searching.

Elsie's daughter always made it clear she liked her mom to get fresh air as often as possible. Over the years Elsie and I took hundreds of walks together. We visited the flower gardens. During our one-sided conversations, I spoke of how impressed I was to see a daughter visit so often. That she must have been a wonderful Mom.

"Can you smell the freshly mowed grass, Elsie? Isn't it sweet?"

I pulled up chairs and we sat by the lake, a place I sensed she enjoyed. There are flower and vegetable gardens, the vegetables planted and tended by residents of Mount View. If we were lucky, we saw a deer or two sneaking past, through the wooded area just beyond the fence. A co-worker once counted eleven, a small herd, trotting by. For a couple of years we had a family of foxes. There were local ducks and geese. The geese usually steered clear, but ducks always waddled around the grounds, splashing in rain puddles and resting on the wet grass. If I ran out of things to say, it didn't really matter. We took in the view together. When we spent time like this, there was no wandering, no searching, no right way or wrong way. Sure I had to watch out for Elsie, but we were not a caregiver and a person living with Alzheimer's.

We were simply two of God's creations, together, getting by as best we could.

One beautiful afternoon I decided to take Elsie for a stroll outside, but first I had to find her. As always, she was wandering. Eventually, I located her in her own room, the last place I thought to look. I extended my hand.

"Elsie, it's gorgeous outside, let's you and me take a walk. I've got stuff I want to talk to you about anyway."

Elsie took my hand, but after a few steps, she stopped. Turning to face me with a voice calm and strong, Elsie spoke for the first time in all the years I'd known her. Her message was short, just three words. But unmistakable, as clear as a Christmas morning.

"I love you."

I can't believe they pay me to do this job!

In the past, I had witnessed the puzzled stares of some patients who seemed to be searching for the purpose of life. My time as a caregiver had led me to a world riddled with roadblocks, countless missteps and seemingly unanswerable questions. Those three words gave meaning to this place and hope for those who doubted. She hasn't spoken since, but it was the moment, and shiver of a lifetime. Elsie had given me the answer, so simple, hiding in plain view all this time. *Love. It's all about love.*

ᕦ ᕤ

I spent nearly seven years working at the nursing home and still attend the funerals for people I knew there.

When Eddie died, I knew it was a service I didn't want to miss. I talked with Eddie's wife and sons on several occasions when they came to visit, though Eddie hadn't been with us all that long before I retired. There were dozens of families I knew better. Still, they were good, down-to-earth people, and Eddie had been more than simply another person I helped care for. He'd been a deer hunting buddy! I *had* to go to his service!

When I arrived, I offered my condolences to Eddie's wife and older son, who were inside the church greeting people. As I was leaving, I bumped into the younger son outside. He seemed completely out of his element, chain smoking and looking about as uncomfortable as a man could get. I guessed his age to be early to mid- thirties, and though I'm six feet tall, he towered over me. He had the look of a lumberjack, or maybe an iron worker. We talked for perhaps a minute, saying things that people who don't know each other that well are supposed to say at funerals. Then, without warning and in mid-sentence, I found myself engulfed in a bear hug. I was forced to hurry for my car. A man's tears should be private.

People always ask, "How could you do that job?"
God Almighty, what a dumb question!

ఌ ఎ

While writing this book and since my retirement several months ago, with one exception, nearly all of my friends on the Unit have died. George, Sid, Eddie, Ned, Elsie, Leona, everyone except Lettie. I was reluctant to describe Lettie in detail. Her issues were so complex and my limitations so numerous I simply didn't feel qualified. This week someone from the nursing home called me. Lettie was not doing well and they figured I would want to know. She had gotten sick to her stomach, had taken to bed, and was not getting up. It appeared she was failing.

I am certain many staff members would agree, of all the residents under our care, no one could be more confusing, confounding, exasperating than Lettie. I'm just as certain that no other resident will be more deeply missed.

I had visited with Lettie a few days before the phone call alerting me to her decline. When she saw me, she began obsessing as always, mad at my wife for not letting me out more. Rather than admitting blame for not visiting as often as she expected, I confessed to her that I was a prisoner of love. We had a good talk.

As I walked to the nursing home to see her for perhaps the final time, my mind recounted some of the outrageous scenarios the two of us had experienced together. How she had "helped" me deliver the Sunday paper to various units throughout the building. Halfway down the hall she decided that the papers were old and needed to be thrown out. *Have you ever attempted to gather up and reorganize half a dozen editions of the Sunday paper?* At our first stop, she refused to let the papers go. At the next stop, she gave them all away. There were times on a cold day when she was hot, and hot days when she claimed to be freezing. There were occasions when she didn't like the other residents and struck out at them, and times when she loved the other residents and refused to eat so they could have her food.

On her worst days, and there were many, getting her into a wheelchair and taking her for a walk was the only solution. No matter what outrageous fiasco she was involved in, she would calm down and go completely silent once seated in her wheelchair and moving. Though God forbid, you stopped for a moment to talk to someone, or to simply catch your breath. The calamity going on before the walk would pale in comparison to what you had on your hands now. I'd spent entire afternoons parading Lettie around the perimeter of the complex. Had I been paid five dollars per loop, I no doubt would have realized a higher tax bracket.

Most of Lettie's clothing had been supplied by the nursing home. As I stepped into her room, I was struck by how few possessions she had. An old, battered family album, the photos inside from decades ago. No family pictures on the wall, the things on her night stand had been donated by staff. She'd be leaving this world bankrupt, and helpless, the same way she'd come in. Lettie's former apartment manager, the Good Samaritan who brought her to us in the first place, wrote an obituary. Lettie's condition steadily worsened, and there was no family to do it.

Lettie's eyes were open as she lay motionless, staring at the wall. Her lips were parted slightly, but she didn't speak. I held her hand and said *The Lord's Prayer* aloud, then talked to her at length about the good old days, and all the fun we'd had. Finally, I leaned over far enough so she could see me and asked, "Do you remember me, Lettie?"

She shook her head slightly and whispered. "No." It was the last time we would ever speak. It would have been nice had she answered yes, but it's a small wound when you realize true stories are seldom perfect. There's no way in hell I'll ever forget Lettie.

In a testament to the facility's commitment to its residents, her funeral service will be held at the nursing home. My album is full and empty, all at the same time. I'm not asking you to feel sorry for poor me. I still have my memories. I am a man of great wealth.

∽ ∾

My nature is to look for the light side of a worst-possible situation. I have tried to reveal the countless instances of humor, wit and pure joy contained within the walls of the nursing home. But I worry about whether I've conveyed just how much these people mean to me. The essence of my message is these helpless individuals, devoid of worldly possessions, stripped of identities, bankrupt in the truest sense, were able to fill my heart. I hope I did the same for them.

I especially hope to help erase the stigma so often attached with Alzheimer's. Human dignity is a birthright that does not end with illness. Alzheimer's is a thief that robs people of their past, strips away their future, and leaves a life unfinished. Yet, inside the walls of a dementia unit, human dignity lives. In an atmosphere which at times defies description, it's the whisper heard over a raised voice, the gentle hand that proves strongest. Deep within the darkness of Alzheimer's will be a caregiver, holding a light and sharing the journey—a guardian of lost souls. No one is judged, and no one walks alone.

From 2000 to 2008, while death rates from other major diseases; heart disease, stroke, breast cancer, prostate cancer, and HIV all dropped, the ratio of deaths from Alzheimer's disease rose sixty-six percent. Until a cure is found, this trend will continue. We already know that certain neurons in the brain die off during early stages of Alzheimer's disease. People don't actually lose their memories, but rather, access to those memories. Recently, researchers at Northwestern University have implanted lab generated cells into mice that produce memory pathways, replicating the work that would have been done by damaged neurons. This effort opens the door to new theories and advanced hope in the battle against Alzheimer's.

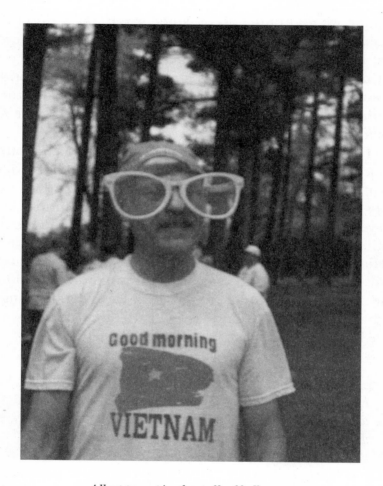

All set to umpire the staff softball game.

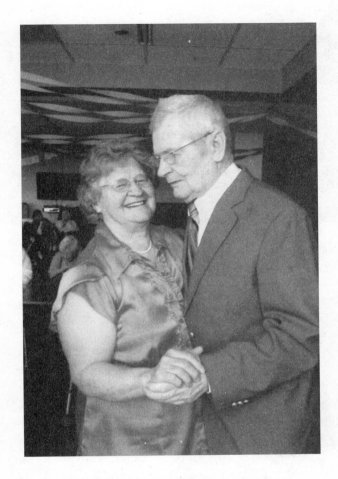

My buddy Ed in his wife's arms—a woman
he eventually referred to as "you."

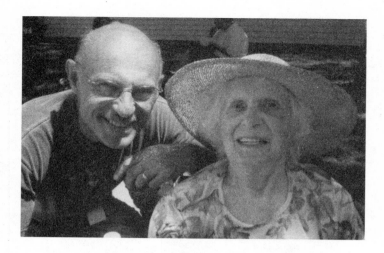

When she came to us, Susan suffered from depression, refusing her
medication. This photo was taken at the Fair.

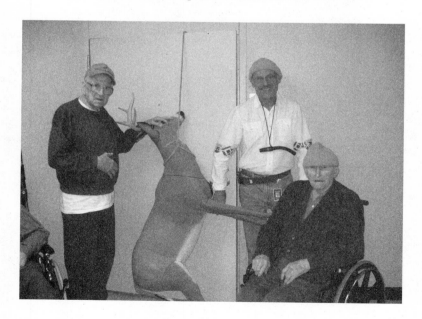

Eddie on the left, with his buck. I guess I'm the guide. The gentleman on the right
was 100 years old when this photo was taken. A final deer season for both men.

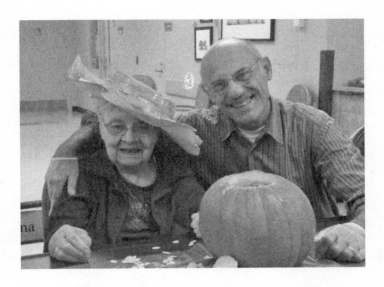

Nora knows things are slipping away.
For twenty-five years she taught Sunday school.

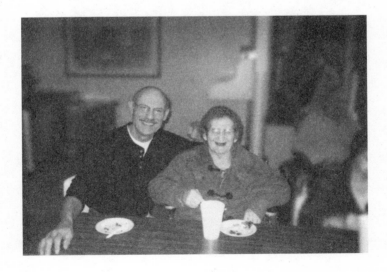

There's no way in hell I'll ever forget Lettie!

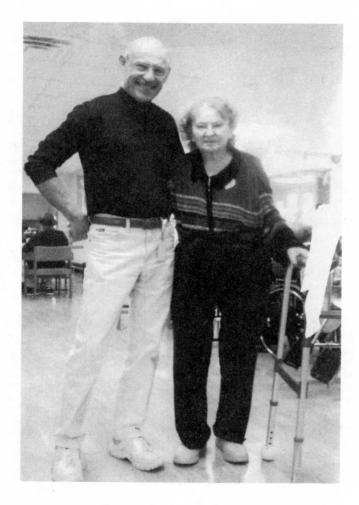

Gertie always asked me what time it was!

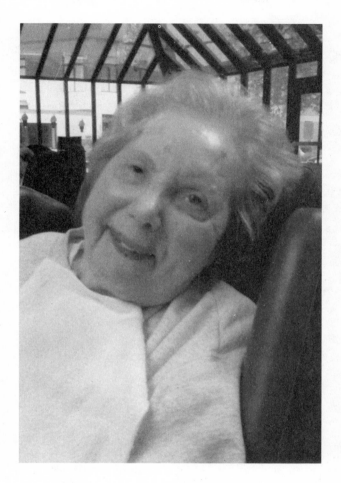

*I've never met a braver heart than
Sally's. I still miss her.*

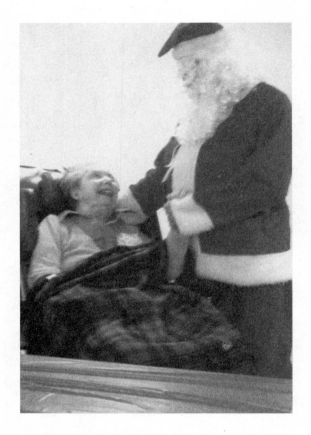

*Sally could only move her head
and her left hand.*

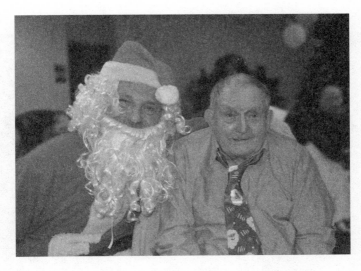

Roy wanted me to get a fire going. He was planning to roast a pig.
One of James Campbell's Ghost Mountain boys, and an American hero.

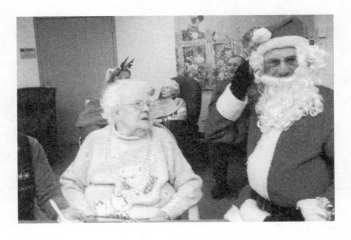

Linda's eyes followed me wherever I went. "We could put on little black hats
and pretend we're typewriters. OH-h-h. NO-o-o."

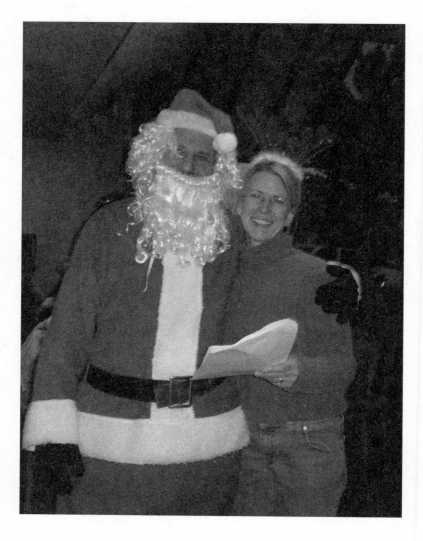

My beautiful wife, Maggie.

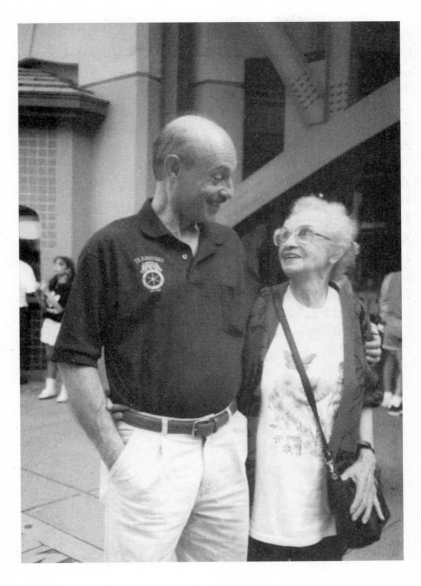

My mother and I.

An Alzheimer's Disease Bill Of Rights.

Every person diagnosed with Alzheimer's disease or a
related disorder deserves:

To be informed of one's diagnosis.

To have appropriate, ongoing medical care.

To be productive in work and play for as long as possible.

To be treated like an adult, not a child.

To have expressed feelings taken seriously.

To be free from psychotropic medications if at all possible.

To live in a safe, structured and predictable environment.

To enjoy meaningful activities to fill each day.

To be out-of-doors on a regular basis.

*To have physical contact including hugging, caressing, and
hand-holding.*

*To be with persons who know one's life story, including cultural
and religious traditions.*

To be cared for by individuals well-trained in dementia care.

INFORMATION ABOUT ALZHEIMER'S DISEASE:
www.alz.org
www.nia.nih.gov/Alzheimers/Alzheimers/information/
generalinfo

PUBLICATIONS:
www.nia.nih.gov/Alzheimers/publications/
browserandorder.htm

CLINICAL TRIALS/RESEARCH:
www.alz.org/trialmatch
www.nia.nih.gov/Alzheimers/researchinformation/
clinicaltrials

[ADEAR] ALZHEIMER'S EDUCATION AND REFERRAL CENTER:
www.nia.nih.gov/Alzheimers/researchinformation/
researchcenter
PHONE 24/7: 1-800-438-4380

CAREGIVING:
www.nia.nih.gov/Alzheimers/caregiving
TheCaregiversVoice.com

Sources

Fisher Center for Alzheimer's Research - www.alzinfo.org
Alzheimer's Association - www.alz.org
National Institute on Aging - www.nia.nih.gov
The Lancet [1997] 349; 1546-1549
Great Short Works of Henry David Thoreau - Harper & Row
[1982] 173
Snapshot- Marathon County Wisconsin - 2009-2011 Edition
American Health Assistance Foundation - www.ahaf.org
Pearls of Wisdom, Jerome Agel and Walter D. Glanze - Harper
& Row [1987] 5, 9, 130
Population: 485 Meeting Your Neighbors One Siren at a Time,
Michael Perry - HarperCollins [2002] 95
Marathon   County   Historical   Society   -   www.
marathoncountyhistory.org
Centers for Disease Control and Prevention - www.cdc.gov/
nchs/fastats/deaths
The Week 3- 25- 2011; 24

Epilogue

In the past decade I've gone from truck driver, to Certified Nursing Assistant, to author, and now speaker and advocate on behalf of our elderly. I might end up giving violin lessons to prison inmates if this keeps up much longer.

In the meantime, I still visit the nursing home regularly. Most days I'm there at noon to assist a lady with her meal. No longer an employee, I'm not allowed to read Annie's background. I have figured out she is Catholic, from the prayer we recite before eating. I'm guessing Annie is in her eighties, and a nurse told me she has no living relatives, only a guardian who seldom visits. Annie suffers anxiety. She asks about her "Papa." *Have I seen him?* It pulls at my heart to see her gripped in fear, clutching her doll. Her baby. Other days she refers to *me* as Papa. I consider it a compliment.

Annie can't remember my name, but she does recognize me when I arrive. As I sit down her face brightens. She puts my hand to her cheek and whispers, "God bless You, God loves you." *Can you imagine how that makes me feel?* It's not important for someone with dementia to know who you are. Knowing you are someone who cares about them is all that matters.

During her meal Annie's hand will reach out, her worn fingers picking at tiny specks, invisible to me. I've noticed this with many dementia patients and have always wondered, *"What in the world is it they see that I cannot?"*

Well, it's finally dawned on me, and no wonder I'm not able to see, because it's something not from this world...angel dust.

The dementia ward taught me not every solution is found within a pill bottle. Not every answer located in a textbook. In CNA class, the nursing home's version of boot camp, it became apparent I would not be able to perform personal cares. My care giving career *could* have ended right then and there, but the facility kept me anyway, with low pay, and a poorly defined job description. Though I had doubts, God's sense of humor led me to what would become the most rewarding time of my life. *I wish every facility would consider creating a position like the one I had.*

A Funny Thing Happened on My Way to the Dementia Ward – Memoir of a Male CNA is now required text in two colleges I'm aware of, for students considering working with the elderly, and has led to an unexpected speaking career. From church basements to fifth floor board rooms, people identify with and embrace the message, and story, of a common man. I don't mention this with hopes of recognition, but to point out we all have gifts to give.

Please consider volunteering at a nursing home. Many provide free classes on basic dementia training. Or contact the Alzheimer's Association for training sites. So very important, because there's an Annie somewhere, gripping her doll, frightened, and waiting for you.

Author Biography

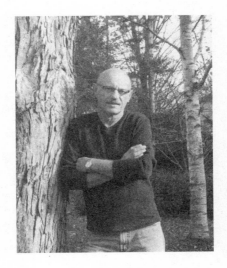

Charles Schoenfeld is a member of Writers of Wausau and the Wisconsin Writers Association. Recently retired, he spends most of his time chasing deer or golf balls.

He is a volunteer with the Alzheimer's Association, Faith in Action, and United Way of Marathon County. He lives in Wausau, Wisconsin with his wife, Maggie. This is his first book.